TOTAL STRETCHING

PHILIP J. TYNE &
MATT MITCHELL

Contemporary Books, Inc.
Chicago

Library of Congress Cataloging in Publication Data

Tyne, Philip J.
   Total stretching.

   Bibliography: p.
   Includes index.
   1. Exercise.   2. Stretch (Physiology)   I. Mitchell,
Matt.   II. Title.
GV505.T96   1983   613.7'1   83-15158
ISBN 0-8092-5567-7

Published by Contemporary Books, Inc.
180 North Michigan Avenue, Chicago, Illinois 60601
Manufactured in the United States of America
Library of Congress Catalog Card Number: 83-15158
International Standard Book Number: 0-8092-5567-7

Published simultaneously in Canada by Beaverbooks, Ltd.
195 Allstate Parkway, Valleywood Business Park
Markham, Ontario L3R 4T8 Canada

To Drs. John L. Beck and Diane Sjostrom, whose professional fields are vastly different but whose separate support, assistance, interest, care, and—most importantly—friendship have been remarkably constant and made it possible for me to be here to produce this book

Matt Mitchell
August 1983

Contents

Acknowledgments

The authors wish to thank: photographer Russ Gilbert, who made this book infinitely more than just another assignment; photographic models Charlotte Gregg Davis, a longtime flight attendant with Pacific Southwest Airlines; Joe Briski, an international hammerthrow competitor; Sharon Courtney, the cover girl who has the special flexibility of a gymnast; Scott Fitzkee, a professional football wide receiver who played in the Super Bowl with the Philadelphia Eagles and later with the San Diego Chargers of the National Football League and the Philadelphia Stars of the United States Football League; the staff of the San Diego Sports Medicine Center; and Lynn McCulla, R.P.T., for her technical assistance.

1

Introduction

Stretching has been around as long as man—and then some. Babies, practically from the time they are settling into the crib for the first time, begin stretching. Most seem to be able to put one leg behind their head with no effort. But as they get older and muscles begin bunching up from growth, that seemingly mindless flexibility starts disappearing, but not irretrievably.

You can regain much of that flexibility, almost regardless of your age. Increased flexibility will make you feel better about your body, more in control. As you use this stronger, more flexible body, you will become less prone to strains, tears, and other common injuries.

Only recently has the importance of flexibility been recognized by medical experts and sports trainers. In the past brute strength was emphasized, and the more subtle contributions of body flexibility were often overlooked.

Except in a few athletic disciplines such as gymnastics and ballet, the use and study of stretching to promote flexibility and diminish the chance of injuries did not start to become popular until the 1970s. It was in professional sports that the change in emphasis was first recognized. Alarmed by muscle tears, such as hamstring injuries that would take a high season toll, professional football teams began to search for better methods of prevention.

As football became the sport of the 1970s in the United States, the professionals wasted no expense in seeking experts who could cut down the injury factor. The result was a move to stretching to increase flexibility and strength and decrease injury. These efforts paid off as athletic performances by the more flexible athletes began to improve measurably.

No longer would pregame exercises consist of jumping jacks and some up-down grass drills to "warm up." Now, teams in various sports approach a game in a more relaxed fashion. The pregame drills include locker-room stretching led by trainers as well as on-the-field exercises that incorporate slow, steady, deep breathing to go with carefully orchestrated muscle-elongating stretches.

Stretches were designed to increase the blood flow to the areas being stretched and to decrease the risk of debilitating muscle pulls. The muscle becomes more elongated, and as a result it has a broad range of natural movement. This is the heart of flexibility, its inner secret. A flexible muscle is relieved from tension and is allowed to achieve the full potential of its natural intended use.

This book will tell you how to stretch in a method never explained to the public before. The "hold-relax" system used in professional sports can be applied to you, too. It will give you freer, more expanded use of your muscles and will help reduce the chances of injury in your everyday life. It works.

Stretching has applications for more than just the professional athlete or occasional jogger. It's an excellent tension reliever for the airline traveler, the deskbound worker, and the housewife who is burdened with numerous household and parental chores.

Almost everyone does some stretching involuntarily. Upon awakening, most people stretch because their bodies just demand such movements before starting the day. Stretching to get rid of tension or muscle stiffness or to prepare for an athletic activity usually requires two segments of self-discipline:

1. remembering to stretch;
2. taking the time to do it.

The most lithe of animals, the cat, never seems to limp around with muscle pulls. The cat probably owes seven of its fabled nine lives to the fact that it's a stretching addict—or at least a fanatic. Watch a cat stretch. Just about every muscle gets involved before it finishes a carefully orchestrated pattern.

While it cannot be guaranteed that stretching will prevent all human muscle pulls or tears, the people who invest the most in trying to eliminate injuries—the sports professionals—have found a remarkable decrease in games missed from torn muscles during the last decade.

Medically there has been a substantial move toward stretching as a method for injury rehabilitation and prevention. Noted knee surgeons are now more apt to prescribe therapy programs that emphasize stretching using proprioceptive neuromuscular facilitation (PNF). PNF focuses largely on range of motion and on strength. This book emphasizes the concept of PNF, which was originally developed through physical therapy studies done of injured and crippled persons in an internationally known rehabilitation center, The Kabat-Kaiser Institute in Vallejo, California, and was later applied in professional sports to prevent injuries. The technique discussed in this book, generally unknown to the general public, can be called most simply *hold-relax*.

Theory of Hold-Relax

The hold-relax method of stretching is based on Herman Kabat's PNF and is widely used in physical therapy and training rooms. It has been tested over the past 10 years and has been shown to be superior to any of the traditional forms of stretching. Many consider it the most efficient method of increasing the range of motion of muscles and connective tissue. It is far superior to the older "active" or "ballistic" forms of exercise, such as Toe Touches, in which quick, repetitive bouncing movements are used to achieve a greater range. Hold-relax also surpasses the "passive" or "static" method of gradually increasing the pressure on the muscle.

Hold-relax incorporates what seems to be just the opposite of what stretching implies. Instead of being stretched directly, the muscle is contracted or "held" for five seconds against a resistance. Then, as it is "relaxed" for five seconds, the opposing or antagonistic muscles will move it gently into a new and broader range.

A Partner Hamstring Stretch is analyzed below to further understanding of the hold-relax technique.

First, the person to be stretched lies down on his back with both legs extended on the floor. The leg to be stretched is brought up in the air to a *point of tightness* in the hamstring. This point is determined when the person first feels the muscle meeting some resistance. It is important that the leg remaining on the floor be kept straight, as this will enhance the stretching. The partner will kneel down and place his shoulder under the heel of the raised leg. The partner is not in this position to push the leg into a new range as is often done in many stretches; he serves as an immovable object, something for the person being stretched to push his leg against. The hold phase begins when the person being stretched attempts to push his leg back toward the floor against the partner's shoulder.

He starts with an easy muscle contraction of the hamstring and slowly builds that contraction to a near maximal effort. At this time, the partner is simply resisting the effort causing an isometric muscle contraction. The near-maximal effort should be held for five seconds. The instant the isometric contraction is completed, the person being stretched moves his leg back toward his head by contracting the opposite or antagonistic muscles, which in this case are the quadriceps and hip flexors (the front of the thigh). This contraction will pull the leg back toward the head and increase the range of motion of the hamstring.

The most difficult point for students of hold-relax to understand is that flexibility is increased by contracting the antagonistic muscle and not by the partner's pushing the leg into a new range. The antagonistic contraction is the key to hold-relax. Contracting the opposite muscle forces the brain to send a signal to the muscle being stretched *to relax*.

Increasing flexibility through the use of neuromuscular facilitation involves two sensory units, the muscle spindle and the golgi tendon organ. The muscle spindle is located in the skeletal muscle; it monitors muscle movements and assists in regulating them. Like the skeletal muscle, the muscle spindle consists of contractile elements that are attached directly to the fibers of the muscle. Thus, when muscles such as the hamstrings are stretched or contracted, the muscle spindle reacts appropriately.

In the example of the Hamstring Stretch, when the hamstring is sufficiently stretched, the muscle spindle senses this stretch and sends a message called *afferent impulses* to the spinal cord. The spinal cord registers this message, processes it, and sends an impulse to the hamstring fibers to contract to unload or relieve the stress on the muscle spindle. Other forms of stretching besides hold-relax are less effective or dangerous because they override the muscle spindle. This can cause muscle tearing, which may be misinterpreted as increased range of motion.

Through the hold-relax method, the muscle spindle allows safe and significant gains in range of motion. The muscle spindle is still facilitated by the stretch of the hamstrings; however, the isometric contraction of the hamstrings demonstrated in the example by the pressure of the leg down into the partner's shoulder relieves the muscle spindle, causing the spindle to relax and adjust to the new increased length of the hamstrings. Furthermore, the contraction of the quadriceps and hip flexors that follows to move the leg up higher facilitates the relaxation of the hamstrings.

Increased muscle relaxation has also been attributed to the golgi tendon organ. This organ, located in the tendons of the muscles, is sensitive to tension caused by both muscle contraction and muscle stretch. During the isometric contraction of the hamstrings the tension may cause the golgi tendon organ to activate, bringing about "inhibition" or relaxation of the hamstrings.

Research on Neuromuscular Facilitation

To date, two studies have been done comparing facilitation stretching with other methods of increasing range of motion. The first study, by Holt, Travis, and Okita (1970), compares the effectiveness of the hold-relax method with the active stretch and static stretching techniques. The purpose of the study was to determine which of the three methods of stretching was most effective in increasing trunk flexion in the long sitting position. Using the sit-reach box, described in Chapter 3, the investigations measured

the amount of improvement each subject gained after participation in one of the three types of stretches. Both feet were kept in
a stationary position and the knees in a completely extended
position lying against the flat surface of the measuring device. The
average increase in range of motion for the static stretch method
was three-fourths of an inch; for the ballistic stretch, slightly less
than three-fourths of an inch; for the hold-relax technique, more
than two inches. That means subjects received nearly three times
the increase in range of motion using the hold-relax technique.

A recent study by Tanigawa (1972) compared the effect of PNF
and passive mobilization on the flexibility of tight hamstring muscles. The results indicated a superiority of the PNF approach in
both increased range of motion and faster rates of improvement.

Due to the success of neuromuscular facilitation techniques and
to research studies that indicate the efficiency of hold-relax
methods, we advocate the use of the hold-relax approach for
anyone striving for excellence in a flexibility program. Improved
performance through greater range of motion, greater muscle
relaxation, and fewer injuries due to tearing of muscle and connective tissue are the benefits that can be derived from this new
approach.

The first time you try it, you will see dramatic results; however,
repeating this over longer periods of time is necessary to maintain
the broadened range. You must follow the instructions in this book
as part of a new commitment to your body if you want to achieve
this free and stronger movement permanently.

WHY STRETCH?

When stretching as a routine entered professional sports it was
envisioned as an injury prevention measure. Soon it became
apparent that it increased the range of motion of joints such as the
hip and the shoulder. Athletic performances also improved. The
overall effects were those of preparing the body for vigorous
activity and increasing circulation in and around muscles and
joints. Athletes realized that tension reduction and muscle relaxation were additional benefits of flexibility exercises.

These benefits need not be limited to athletes. What person with a desk job who experiences a painfully tight neck or a housewife with an ache in her low back from vacuuming would not want or need exercises that would help decrease the discomfort? By performing regular flexibility exercises you may free yourself from daily discomfort due to tight muscles and poor posture.

Stretching can be done almost everywhere and anytime. It requires no special equipment. You can be standing, sitting, or lying down. It works sitting behind a desk or in the car or on a long airline trip.

There is probably no time not to stretch, but there are periods when stretching should be done.

- before starting any strenuous physical activity
- after long periods of inactivity, including sitting, standing, or driving
- when you feel tired or tense
- when finishing an activity to help keep muscle fibers elongated

A few terms used frequently in this book are defined below.

Flexibility—the maximum range of motion possible for any joint.

Isometric—contracting a muscle against an immovable force.

Range of motion—the number of degrees of arc a joint can travel.

Strength—the maximum effort that can be produced in one movement.

Elongate—to increase the length of a muscle.

Agilities—rapid movements and change of directions which prepare the body for a particular activity.

Rotations—movements which increase the fluid in a joint.

Static stretching—using gradual pressure to increase the muscle's range of motion.

WHAT TO EXPECT?

Flexibility doesn't occur instantly. It's taken a lot of years for most people to become stiff and relatively rigid, so it will take time to become flexible again.

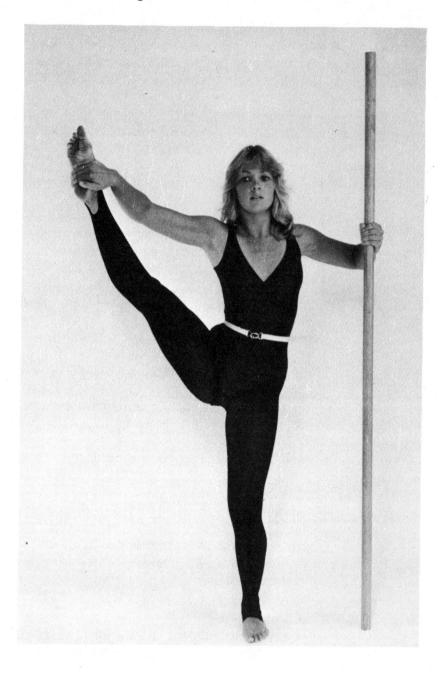

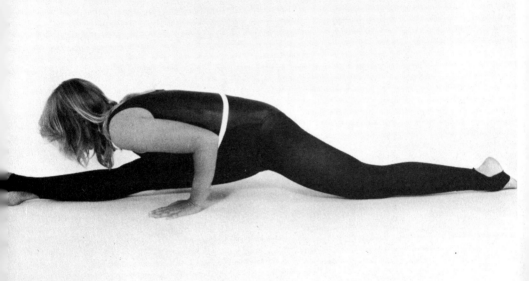

Don't be discouraged by apparent setbacks. The body seems to experience periods of improvement, then minor losses before improving again. Also, not everyone is going to become as flexible as a gymnast, who can do splits, or a ballet dancer, who has no trouble raising a foot above her head. Sometimes stretching improvement is delayed simply by muscle fatigue. Do a light stretching routine and don't worry. Within a few days you'll be back on the path to further improvement.

There are various methods of stretching. You may choose to stretch all by yourself or with a partner.

For the less limber, sometimes it is necessary to use a bath towel looped over a foot or ankle to perform the needed stretch. Otherwise, you may not be able to perform an exercise efficiently.

Apparatus such as a cable and pulley with the pulley attached to a fence, pole, door handle, or wall will aid in stretching (see Chapter 9). Having several is invaluable to a team with limited staff or to a person without a partner.

2
The Don'ts and Do's of Stretching

THE DON'TS

1. Don't bounce.

Watch joggers loosen up a bit before going off for a run. Many will stand with feet together and knees rigid, attempting to touch their toes. Each time their hands get close to their feet, they "bounce" a bit, trying to increase their range of motion in their hamstrings and lower back.

This tugging can lead to torn ligaments and microscopic tears in the muscles. Bouncing will cause the muscle to shorten as a defensive measure rather than elongate over time, which is one of the purposes of stretching.

2. Don't push when in pain.

It's macho, of course, to prove how far you can continue despite the pain of a torn muscle or strained tendon or ligament. It's also stupid and will only delay improvement and eventual good health.

11

Pain doesn't mean progress. It's Mother Nature's signal that something's amiss and should be recognized as a danger signal.

3. Don't force your body into a new range of motion.

It sometimes is easy to want to ignore warnings against overstretching. Your body's excellent neuromuscular system will tell you when enough is enough, but it's all too easy to ignore the alarm and go on "just a bit farther."

When working with a partner it's even easier to allow your counterpart to "stretch" you. When you override the built-in controls, you also enhance the opportunity to be set back in a flexibility program due to injury to the muscle. A partner should assist, but not stretch, you.

The method of stretching a muscle is important. A few common stretches that have been demonstrated over and over on television exercise programs or by behind-the-times coaches are potentially injurious. They include the Hurdler's Stretch, the Plow, the Toe Touch, and the Leg-Up Stretch.

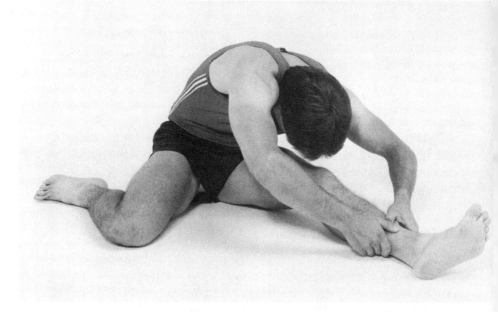

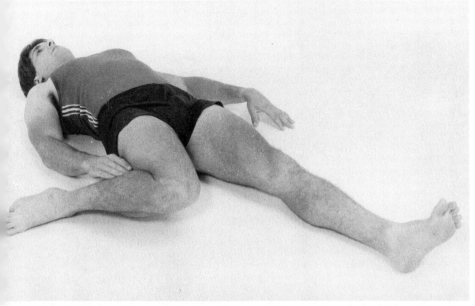

The bent knee in the so-called Hurdler's Stretch quickly becomes suscepti-ble to strains and even torn ligaments from the awkward position. The knee was not meant to be twisted in this way, but some will try to force themselves into the position because they've seen very flexible athletes perform the exercise to stretch their hamstrings (as in photo on page 12) or their thighs (above). A better stretch is done while seated with one knee bent, placing the foot on the opposite thigh. This will allow the hamstring of the straight leg to be stretched without placing undue pressure on the knee joint.

The Plow is a favorite of many, but it compresses the vertebrae in the neck, stretches the ligaments of the entire spine, and can do permanent damage to the back. The back can be stretched more safely by rolling your body into a ball.

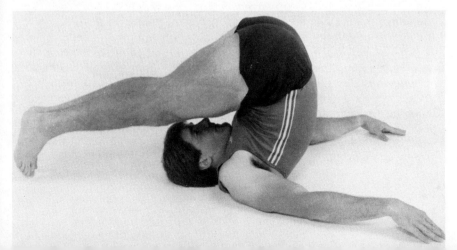

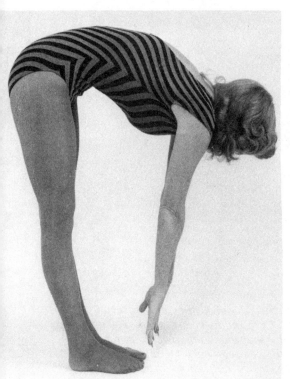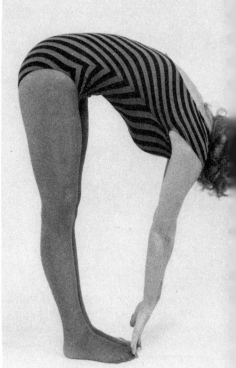

Many people like to touch their toes to demonstrate how flexible they are or as an exercise. However, this exercise is an inefficient method of stretching because the position of standing, with knees straight, causes the muscles of the legs and back to contract to hold the body up. Therefore, stretching this way amounts to attempting to stretch already contracted muscles, which can strain the hamstring and back. Also, toe touching after prolonged sitting or bending may result in the exclamation, "Oh, my back; I can't straighten up." The preferred method for standing stretches involves bending forward with the knees slightly bent to reduce back strain.

For dance students, the bar is used routinely for stretching (as in photo on the next page). This method of stretching the hamstrings can impart tremendous damage to the knee joint because, as the leg is forced to straighten by the upper body weight, the unsupported knee is severely stressed. Cruciate ligaments, cartilages, and other parts of the knee have been injured by this type of stretching. Hold-relax Hamstring Stretches, both straight-leg and bent-knee, will allow one to elongate the muscles safely and efficiently.

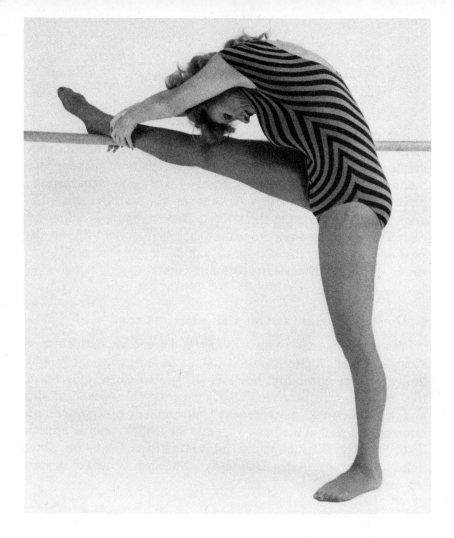

THE DO'S

1. Do feel the stretching in the middle of the muscle.

If it's felt near the end of the muscle being worked on, it's liable to be a ligament or tendon that is being attacked; a strain or tear may result.

2. Do see a doctor before leaping into a strenuous flexibility program.

This is especially important if you've had a history of injuries to joints or the lower back.

3. Do use ice rather than heat on sore or injured areas.

This applies both before and after exercising or competition. Major league baseball, which always has been slow to adapt to new methods of training, has long used ice on pitchers' arms, which has helped lengthen many careers. Notice on television that when a player is injured you'll almost always see him on the bench with a giant ice pack applied to the injured area to reduce swelling and pain. This ice is used not only at the time of injury but should also be used continually throughout the rehabilitation program. Heat is rarely used in a professional training room.

4. Do stretch before and after an exercise period.

Prestretching may reduce injury and improve performance. Most activities, ranging from golf and tennis to running and weightlifting, require flexibility; however, they also cause muscles to tighten. Therefore, poststretching is necessary to regain flexibility and will reduce next-day soreness. Unfortunately, poststretching is often overlooked in the haste to leave the locker room or athletic field. The body is usually warm after athletic participation, which helps loosen the muscles and increase the effectiveness of stretching exercises.

3
Testing for Flexibility

Because everyone's physiology is different, it's impossible to say that each person should have so many degrees of flexibility. It's not like playing golf, where par has been established ahead of time for everyone. Everyone has a separate flexibility scale. But there are methods of testing the flexibility of the major areas of the body. You can make a chart to keep a record of your progress. Don't expect to achieve long-range goals in the short term. Checking about every three months can provide some startling results. All that is needed is a ruler, yardstick, or tape measure. The hamstrings, lower back, abdominal muscles, hip flexors, shoulders, and groin can be measured to establish a bench mark from which improvement can be observed. Remember you should work to improve your own flexibility and not to compare your flexibility with someone else.

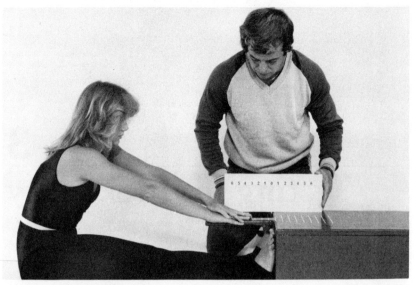

The scale on the sit-reach box shows how tight many people are in the hamstrings when they begin a flexibility program (above). This is a simple wooden box about 10 inches high with a stick that protrudes backward to show negative flexibility. The model would be a minus three inches.

With feet flat against the end of the box and knees out straight (below), Sharon demonstrates her flexibility by being a plus six inches while reaching and trying to keep her back as straight as possible and her knees locked. Hands overlap with fingers touching as she reaches as far as possible.

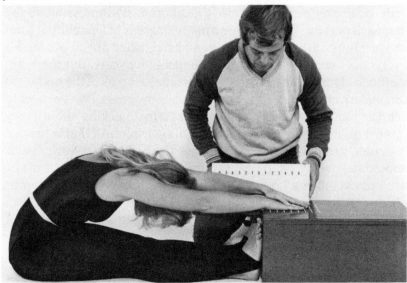

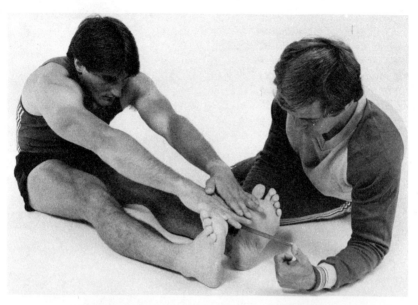

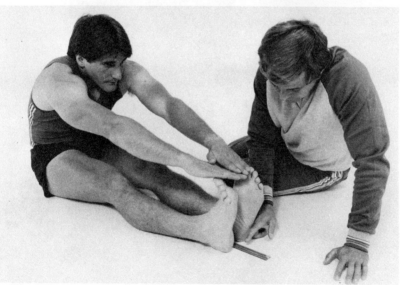

Absent a sit-reach box, a ruler can be used. Put it so the six-inch mark is between the heels, either held by a partner or flat on the floor. Keep the legs flat on the floor, knees locked, with feet as close together as possible and hands overlapping. Simply lean forward and drop the finger onto the ruler.

How flexible is your lower back? One way to measure this is to lie flat on the floor, pull one knee to your chest and measure from the bottom of the breastbone to the top of the kneecap (right). The fewer the inches, the more flexible.

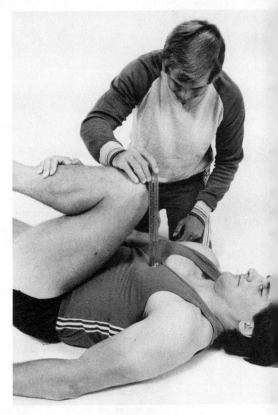

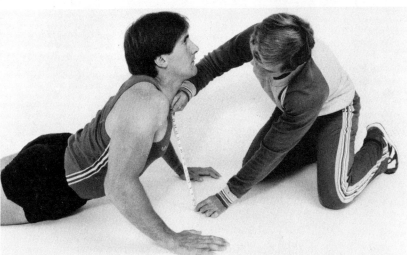

To assess the amount of abdominal flexibility, do a Press-Up while keeping your pelvis on the floor. Measure with a tape from the top of the breastbone directly to the floor.

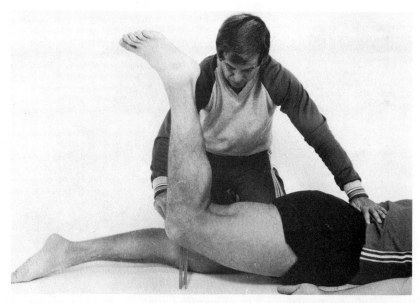

The hip flexors are checked while lying in a facedown position (above). The pelvis must remain flat. Then lift your knee off the floor as far as possible without lifting the pelvis. Measure from the ground to the top of the kneecap. Each leg should be measured since there can be some difference between the two.

For chest and shoulder flexibility, lie facedown on the floor and grasp a ruler or stick between your hands. Keeping your head down, raise the stick as high as possible. Measure the distance from the stick to the floor.

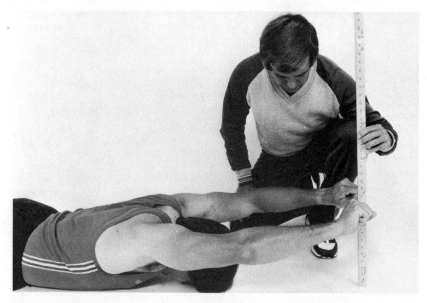

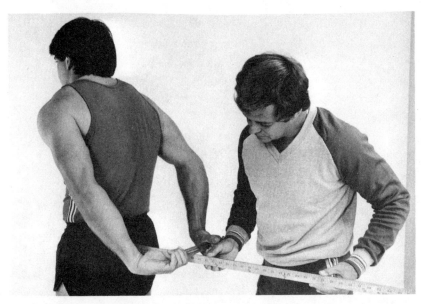

For an additional test for shoulder flexibility (above), stand and hold the stick behind you. Then raise it backward as far as possible. The measurement is made from the tailbone to the stick.

Groin tears are common, especially among people who run and jump. Legs are spread as far apart as possible while keeping them flat on the floor. Measurement is made from the inside of each kneecap.

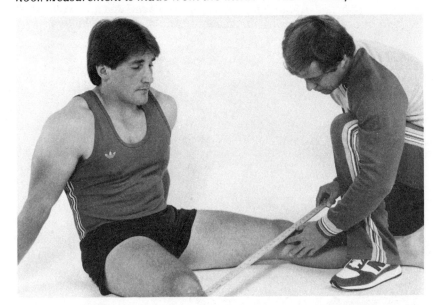

4
Warm-Ups

In order to prepare the body for vigorous activity or for a short run you must first warm up the muscles and lubricate the joints. Performing stretching exercises will do neither. Many people get confused when comparing warming up to stretching. What's the difference? First, warming up should always precede stretching. Warming up is the actual heating up of the body by directly increasing the body's temperature. This increased temperature is accomplished by pumping blood into the muscles and also stimulating the release of synovial fluid (the body's lubricant) into the joints.

A cold muscle can be compared to a dry leaf found on the ground on a fall day. Any attempt to manipulate the leaf results in small tears and cracks. A muscle that is fully pumped with a fresh supply of blood is more like the healthy green leaf picked from the tree in spring; the leaf can be bent and wadded up in your hand, yet it springs back to its original shape without a single tear.

What actually happens inside the body following a warm-up session?

1. For each additional degree of body heat, the cells' metabolic rate increases about 13 percent.
2. Muscles work faster and relax faster.
3. Greater efficiency is achieved because of lower resistance in muscles.
4. Hemoglobin, which carries oxygen in the blood, gives up more oxygen at higher temperatures.
5. The body's metabolism increases.

The important conclusion here is that proper warm-up followed by proper stretching *can improve performance* and may help prevent injuries. The heating of the body can be accomplished by actually exercising, by jogging at a slow pace, by riding a bicycle (stationary or two-wheeler), by jumping on a trampoline, or by jumping rope. Actually any activity that makes you perspire can be considered a warm-up. When you start to perspire, or when you feel an elevated temperature, then it's time to start stretching. An important lesson to remember is that the warm-up is intended only to increase the body temperature; it is not the race, it is not a competition, so set your own pace to get warm. Ten to fifteen minutes of very light movements should be enough to get you ready to start stretching.

The following is a suggested sequence to follow if you want to prepare properly for an athletic event. If you simply want to achieve the benefits of a daily stretching routine, then do the first four. The more strenuous the sport or activity, the more important it is to follow the entire sequence.

1. Warm-up (jogging, jumping rope, bicycling, step-ups, trampoline)
2. Rotations (movement which increases the fluid in the joint)
3. Static stretching (stretches using gradual pressure to increase the range of motion of the muscles)
4. Hold-relax (stretches using the PNF method of isometrically contracting a

muscle, then relaxing and moving to a
new range of motion)
5. Agilities (rapid movements and change
of directions to ready the body for a particular event)
6. Skill rehearsal (throwing the ball,
running, swinging the racquet, catch-
ing, etc.)
7. Participation in the sport
8. Restretching with the hold-relax technique
9. Cool-down (walking to prevent blood
from pooling)

Two of the most overlooked areas are those of restretching after
an activity and the cool-down. Studies have shown that the great-
est improvements in flexibility can be achieved if you do some
stretching exercises after vigorous activity. It stands to reason that
the body is at its highest temperature level immediately after
exercise. So take a few minutes to stretch those legs and back after
your sets of tennis or following that 10k run.

After five minutes of postexercise stretching, walk around and
allow your body to return slowly to its normal temperature. Also
concentrate on relaxing and breathing. This cool-down period is
very important, because it prevents the blood from pooling in the
legs and helps the body return to a state of normal circulation and
body temperature.

JOINT ROTATIONS

Here are five rotational moves that should follow the warm-up
period to help the body get ready for more strenuous activities.
These will elevate the body's temperature at specific points, which
means that more blood is flowing through the muscle structure
and the synovial fluid that lubricates the joints will be more active.
Overall, this is not unlike warming the motor oil in a car in cold
weather before starting out on a high-speed drive.

Also following are some demonstrations with a broom handle
which aid in some shoulder and trunk rotation and also begin some
preliminary stretching of the upper body.

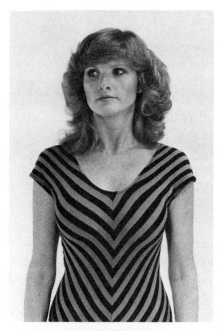
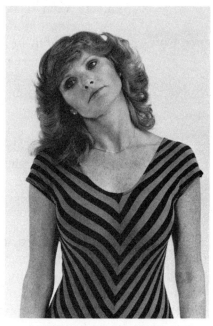

Start with a neck rotation to initiate a loosening-up routine. Turn the head from side to side, rolling it deeply in front. But don't roll it backward because this can cause the neck vertebrae to grind and possibly do some damage over a long period. With each dozen rotations, try to reach a little more to each side and go deeper into the chest.

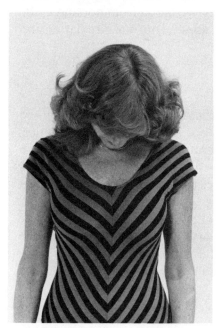
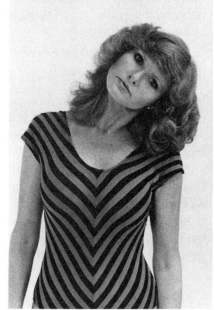

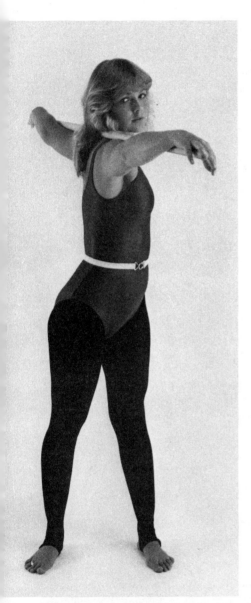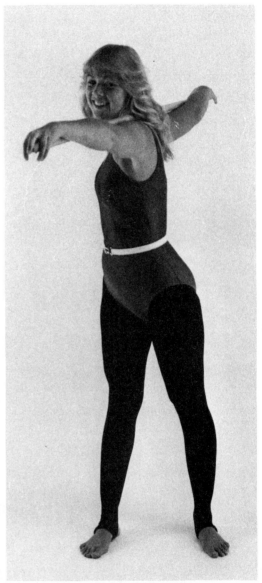

With a pole or broom handle along the top of the shoulders, extend your arms to the side as far as possible. When you are more flexible, the pole can be held across the shoulder blades. Turn slowly from side to side with good, upright posture and a slight bend in the knees. Do it slowly. This is a warm-up, not a world-level competition. Do about 20 turns to each side.

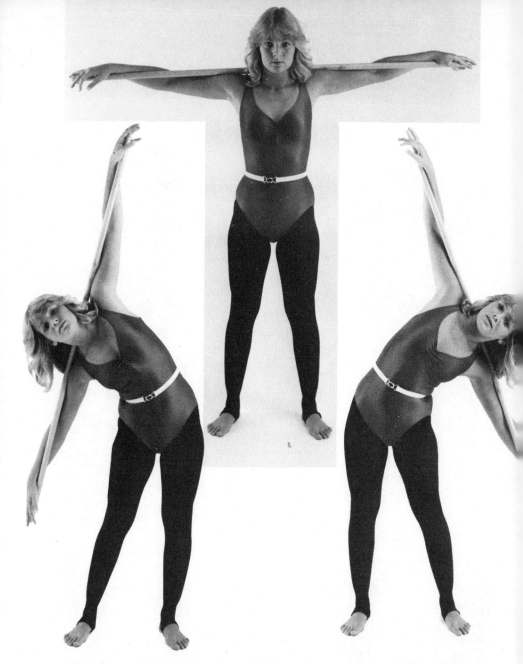

Use the same starting position with the stick as in the preceding twisting routine. Only this time, reach as far to each side as possible. You'll feel a gradual loosening in the side muscles. Maintain good posture by not bending forward at the waist throughout the routine of 12-20 bends to each side. Bending and twisting the trunk (as on page 29) is for the more advanced. It should follow the regular upright twisting warm-up routine. The stick should be held a bit lower so that it doesn't rub against the neck vertebrae. Ten to 20 side-to-side bends are sufficient.

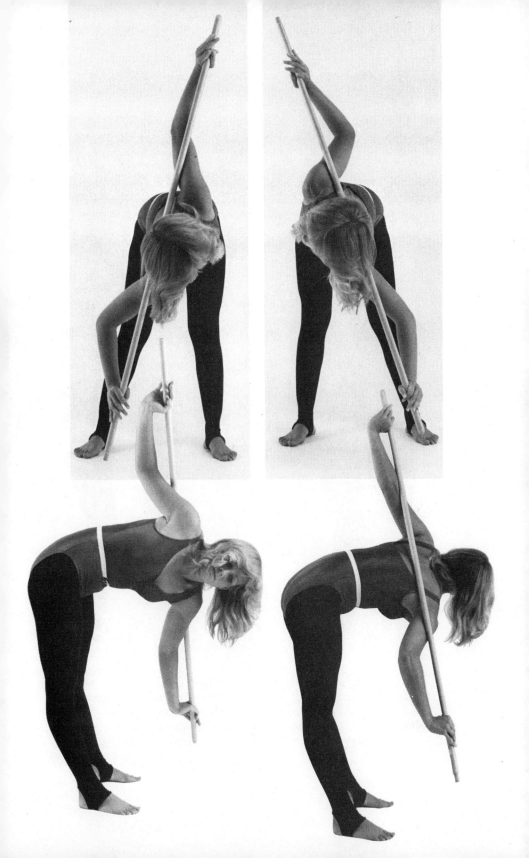

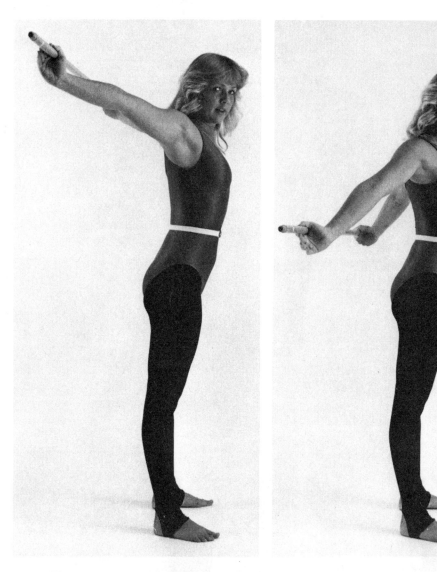

The stick can be used to loosen the shoulders in a very simple exercise. Hold it at arm's length behind you, then drop your arms as far as possible. Advanced athletes with flexible shoulders may be able to hold the stick against their hips in front and, in one slow, fluid move, take it over their heads and continue all the way to the back until it touches their buttocks.

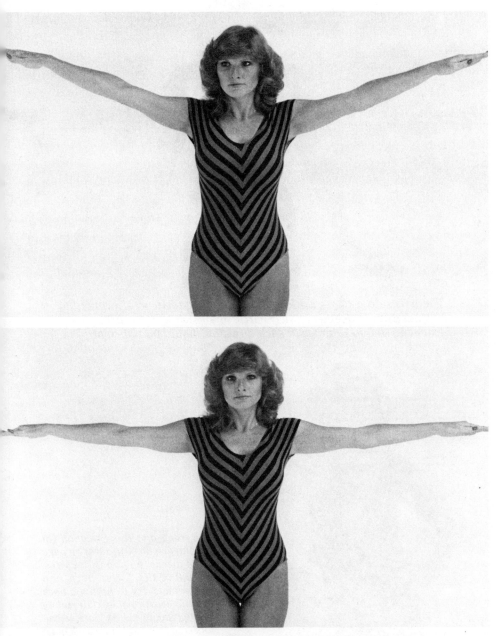

This is a simple routine not unlike the ones children use when playing airplane. But don't rev up your propellers very rapidly. Keep the arms straight and concentrate on rolling the shoulders. Ten slow rotations each way provide a good warm-up.

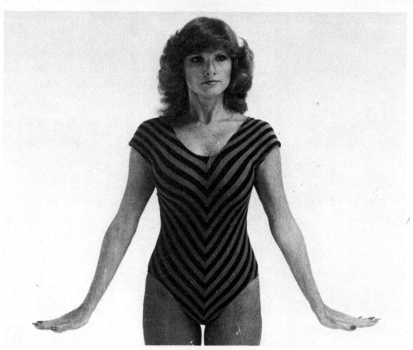

The wrists do a lot of work in most athletic endeavors. Keeping fingers extended and together, slowly circle them while your arms are fully extended. Ten to 12 times in each direction should be sufficient.

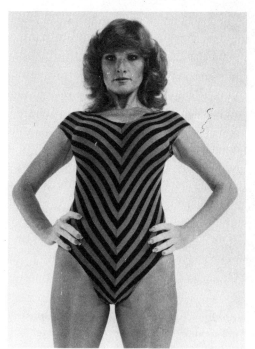

The trunk and torso rotation (at left and first three pictures on page 33) loosens up many muscles, including the lower back and abdominals. Try to keep the back as straight as possible while rolling through the twists. As you become looser, it is possible to stretch out a bit farther with each of the 12 rotations. Do six in one direction before switching to the other direction.

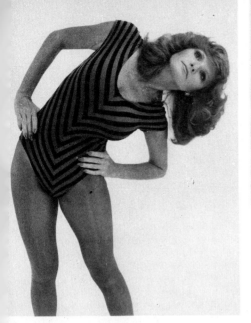
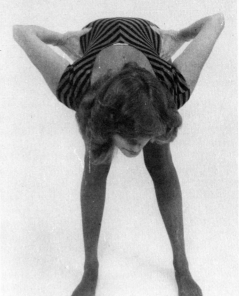
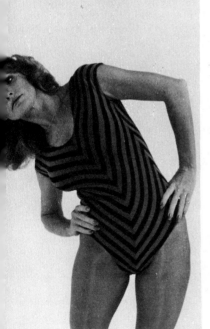
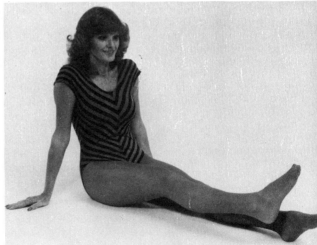

Sit on the floor and extend your legs. Pick up one leg and rotate the ankle six times in one direction, then six in the other. Rotate both ankles before quitting.

5

Methods of Stretching

Once you have warmed up to increase the temperature of the muscles and performed the joint rotations to increase the lubrication around the joints, it is time to choose one of several methods of stretching or elongating the muscle fibers. Stretching exercises can be performed in any of three popular ways: (1) *actively* or *ballistically*; (2) *passively* or *statically*; (3) *hold-relax* method.

Ballistic stretching, which is not recommended, consists of a series of bouncing movements designed to increase the range of motion of a muscle. You have probably seen this form of stretching when a person stands with knees locked, leans forward to touch the toes, and then does a series of bounces or bobbing movements in an attempt to reach farther. These *active* movements can cause damage to the muscles and actually shorten them.

Static stretching involves increasing the length of the muscle without bouncing or forcing. It is simply moving until you feel tightness in the muscle and then holding that position for a given period of time. An example is sitting on the ground with the legs spread, reaching forward as far as you can, and then, when you feel tightness behind your legs, holding that position for 20–30 seconds. Static stretching will increase your flexibility and is used successfully by most athletes.

Hold-relax is a new and more scientific approach to stretching. It involves contracting the muscle and then moving it into a new range while it is relaxed. An example: Lie on your back and raise your right leg in the air. With the leg straight, reach up and grasp the leg with both hands behind the calf. Pull the leg into your hands as if you are attempting to put your heel back on the ground. Hold this isometric contraction for five seconds, then relax and bring the leg closer toward your head.

This book consists of a combination of static and hold-relax stretching routines. Choose exercises that best fit your lifestyle and have fun stretching.

6

Static Stretches for
One Person

Learn to stretch by yourself even if you currently have access to a trainer or partner with whom you can work. There will be times when you should stretch before an activity and there will not be anyone around who is qualified to work with you.

As you become an experienced stretcher and have gained a desired measure of flexibility, you will probably begin to incorporate minor variations into the following suggested exercises. Your body, as it becomes accustomed to the stretching routines, will quickly emit signals that the variations are good or bad. If in doubt, seek out a coach, trainer, or physical therapist who is knowledgeable about flexibility and stretching.

Do the following exercises slowly, deliberately, rhythmically, and under control to gain the best results. This can be accomplished more easily using a pause-and-relax routine as often as is feasible. If nothing else, incorporating a pause makes it harder to bounce. During static-type stretching each new position should be held for approximately 30 seconds to allow the muscle to adjust to its new length.

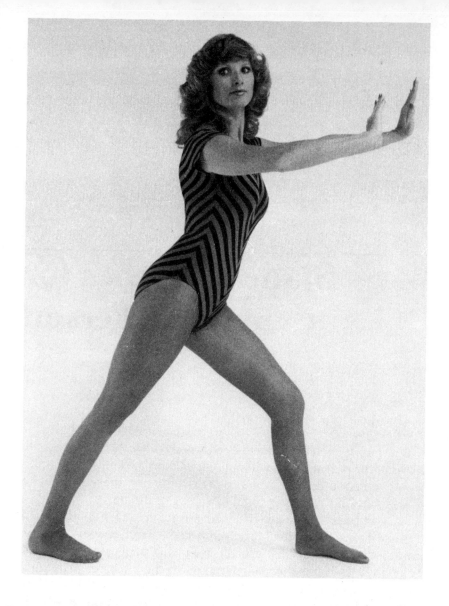

Calf and Achilles Tendon

You'll feel immediate results from the easy exercise shown above. Lean against a solid object, both feet straight in line with the weight over the front foot. The back should be kept straight. Most importantly, keep the back heel flat on the ground.

Push the back heel into the ground while leaning forward.

To increase the stretch, lean forward.

Pause in each repetition and exhale. Do six repetitions, then switch and use the other leg for six. Each position should be held for 30 seconds.

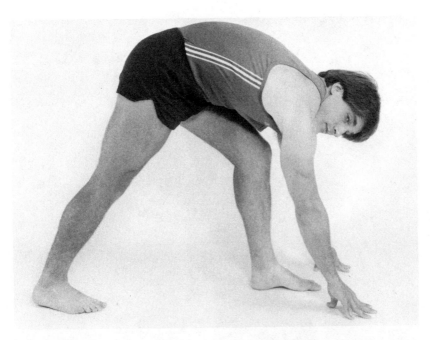

With both feet pointed straight ahead, step forward about a foot and a half with the left leg, then bend over and attempt to touch the ground with the fingertips. Keep the bulk of the body weight over the front leg and keep the back heel flat on the ground. Push the back heel back on the ground.

To increase the stretch, lean the weight forward a bit more and even step forward slightly.

Pause after each repetition and exhale. Do six repetitions, then switch and use the other leg for six.

Shin

Don't wait until you have "shin splints" to stretch out the shin muscles. In the same position as for the Upright Calf and Achilles Tendon Stretch, lean against a wall or a solid object with the left leg in front of the right, as seen on the following page. In this case, however, the right foot is arched backward so that the top of the toes are touching the ground.

Push the right foot against the ground while leaning forward. To increase the stretch, lean forward more and step slightly farther forward with the left leg.

Pause after each repetition and exhale. Do six repetitions, then switch and use the other leg for six.

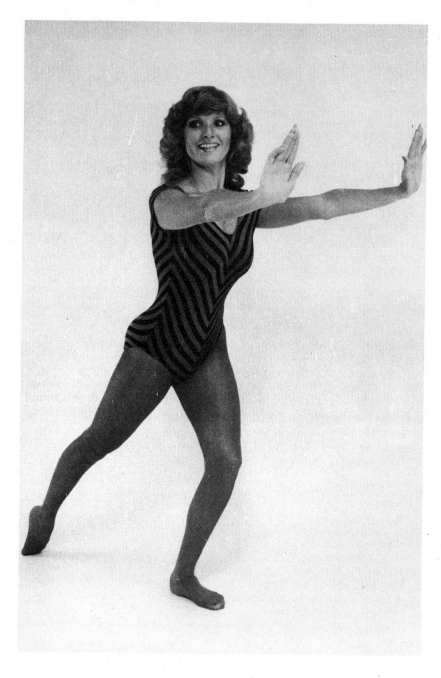

Hamstrings

This stretch immediately helps you locate the hamstrings if you're not sure where they are.

Stand with legs slightly farther apart than shoulder width, bend both knees and bend over at the waist. Place both hands flat on the floor. Then slowly raise your hips and back while keeping your hands flat on the floor. If the legs straighten easily, then bend over again and move the hands back toward the feet.

Pause after each repetition and exhale. Do six repetitions. Remember to hold the stretch for 30 seconds.

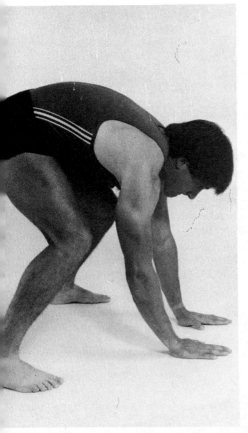
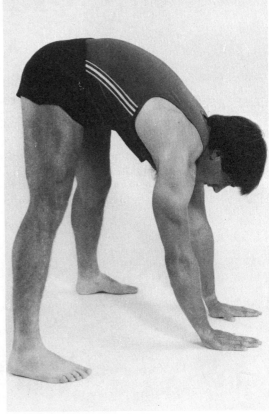

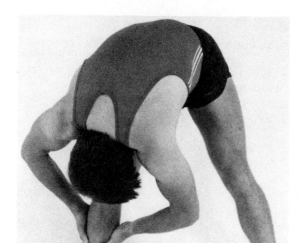

Stand up straight with legs spread farther apart than shoulder width, then bend over and grasp the right calf with both hands and touch your head to the kneecap (left). Pause and exhale. Stand up, then bend over and repeat the exercise, attempting to touch the head closer to the kneecap or farther down the shin.

Do six repetitions, then switch to the other leg for six.

Lie flat on the ground, bring your right leg to your chest, and place both hands behind the knee across the hamstring muscle (below).

Then attempt to straighten the leg as far as possible (top of page 43). Keep the left leg as flat as possible throughout this routine. Bend the knee, then attempt to straighten it again. Pause after each repetition and exhale. Do six repetitions, then switch to the other leg for six. Don't be discouraged if you cannot straighten your leg completely. In order to stretch the hamstring, the knee must be kept close to the chest, and this should prevent the leg from being completely straightened.

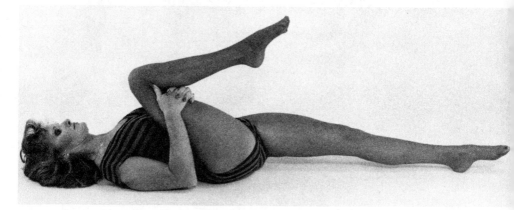

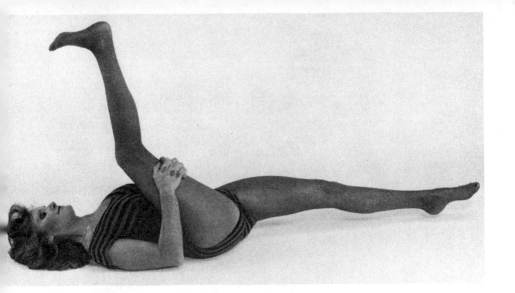

Sit flat on the floor and spread both legs as far apart as is comfortable (below). Then reach forward as far as possible. Pause for 30 seconds when you have attained the limit of your reach, sit back up, then repeat the exercise. Do six repetitions.

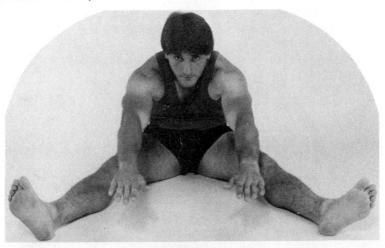

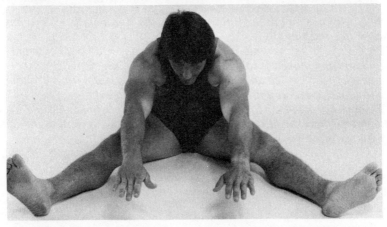

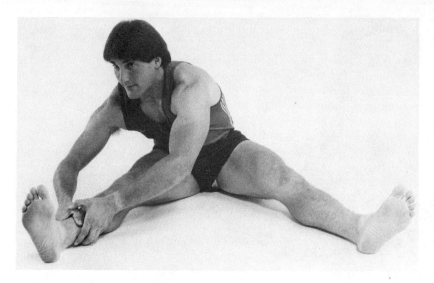

The exercise shown above stretches not only the hamstrings but also the low back.

Sit with legs spread as far apart as is comfortable. Keeping both legs flat on the ground, reach out and attempt to grasp the ankle, calf, or area of the leg near the knee. Attempt to lower your head toward your kneecap. Pause and exhale. To increase the stretch, lean farther forward.

Do six repetitions, then switch to the other leg for six.

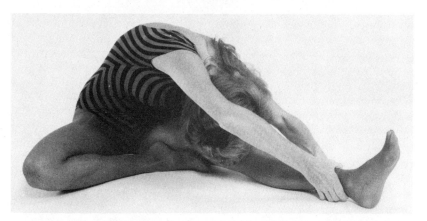

This stretch is an excellent substitute for the Hurdler's Stretch (a major "don't" in stretching).

Sit with both legs spread as far apart as is comfortable. Then bend the right knee and place the sole of the right foot against the inner part of the left thigh. Grasp the left ankle with both hands and lean forward, attempting to touch your head to the kneecap. Pause and exhale.

Sit back up, then lean forward. Grasp farther down the ankle and again attempt to touch the kneecap. Do six repetitions, then switch to the other leg for six.

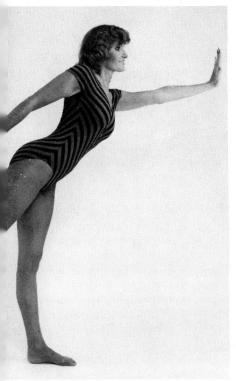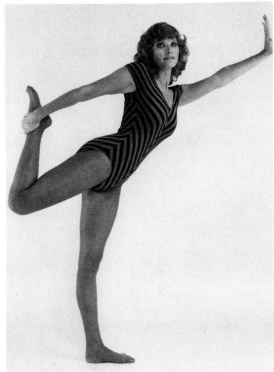

Thighs
(Quadriceps)

Stand with the left hand against a wall, then raise the right leg back as far as possible, bending at the knee (above). Grasp the right ankle with the right hand and hold the right leg upward, attempting to raise the knee farther from the ground. Pause and exhale.

Raise the knee even farther from the ground to increase the stretch.

Do six repetitions, then switch to the other leg for six.

Try the stretch shown at the top of page 46 if you're too stiff or muscular to reach your ankle with ease.

Lie facedown, flat on the floor. Raise the right leg off the ground and bend the knee as far as possible. Grasp the right ankle with the right hand, then attempt to raise the leg farther from the floor. Pause and exhale.

Raise the knee even farther from the ground to increase the stretch.

Do six repetitions, then switch to the other leg for six. If you cannot grasp the ankle with your hand, take a towel and wrap it around the ankle and hold the ends of the towel to do this exercise.

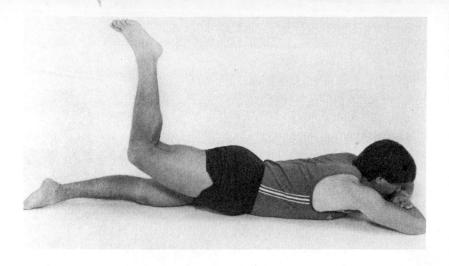

Lie down on your left side, then raise the right leg and bend the right knee as far as possible (below). Grasp the right ankle with the right hand and gradually attempt to touch the heel to the buttocks.

Pause and exhale.

Pull the leg and foot farther toward the buttocks to increase the stretch.

Do six repetitions, then switch to the other leg for six.

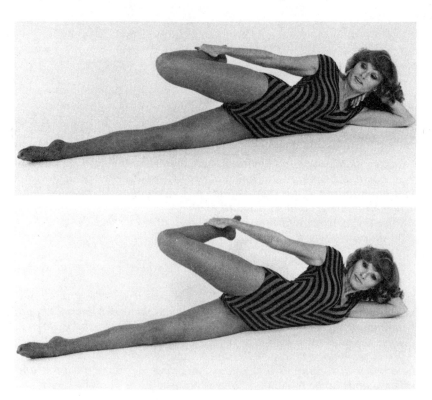

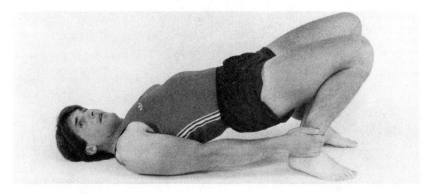

Lie flat on your back on the floor, then bend your knees as much as possible, pulling your feet in under your body (above). Grasp your ankles with both hands. Rise up and arch your back. Do not arch your neck.

Pause and exhale. Then pull the ankles even farther under the body and repeat the exercise. Do six repetitions. Beware of arching your neck!

Groin

Stand up straight, then spread your legs as far apart as possible. Turn the left leg and attempt to stride away while leaving the right foot stationary (below). Most of the body weight is over the left side as the left foot points away from the right foot. Push the right foot into the ground while leaning forward over the left foot.

To increase the stretch, lean farther forward over the left foot. Pause after each repetition and exhale. Do six repetitions, then switch to the other leg for six.

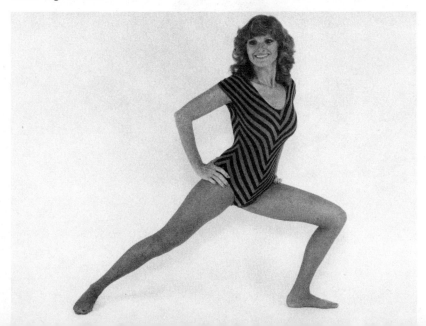

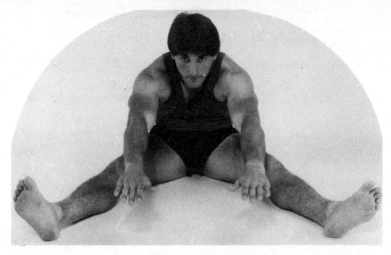

Sit on the ground with legs spread as far apart as possible. Reach forward toward an imaginary target (above). Keep the back as straight as possible. To increase the stretch, sit back up and then lean farther forward. Also, spread the legs farther apart with each repetition. Pause after each repetition and exhale. Do six repetitions.

Sit on the floor with spine straight and pull the heels together and as close to the body as possible. Hold the feet in both hands, then lean forward (below).

To increase the stretch, pull the feet even closer to the body and open the knees farther so that they are closer to touching the floor.

Pause after each repetition and exhale. Do six repetitions.

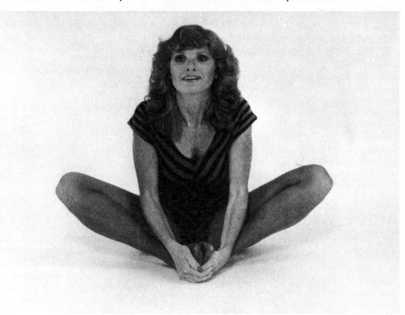

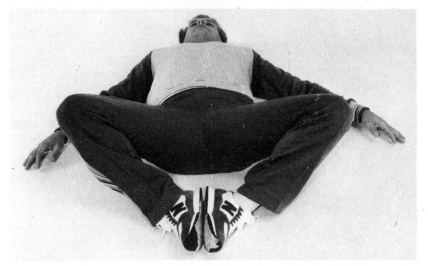

Lie flat on the floor and place the soles of your feet together. Bend both knees and pull your feet as close to your body as possible. Spread your arms out to the sides. Allow the knees to drop closer to the floor.

To increase the stretch, pull the feet slightly closer to the body and drop the knees even closer to the floor.

Pause after each repetition and exhale. Do six repetitions.

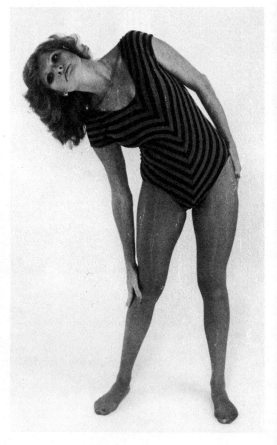

Side Stretches (Obliques)

Stand up straight. Then, keeping the head and body in good posture, bend directly to the side, trying to touch as far down your leg as possible. First do the stretch to the right side, touching the right hand to the outside of the right knee. Then stand up straight and reach to the left side, touching the left knee. With each repetition, you should be able to touch farther down the leg. Feet will be kept at shoulder width and pointed straight ahead. Do not bend forward at the waist.

Pause after each repetition and exhale. Do six repetitions on each side.

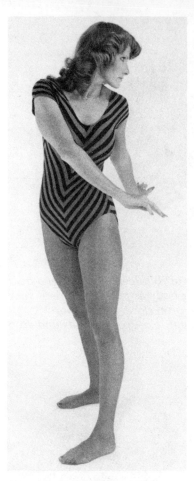

Standing straight with feet parallel and pointed straight ahead (left), slowly turn to one side, reaching behind you as far as possible with both hands. Your hips and pelvis should remain as straight as possible during this exercise. The stretch is effected by turning at the sides and upper body.

To increase the stretch, reach farther behind you each time. Pause after each repetition and exhale. Do six repetitions alternately to each side.

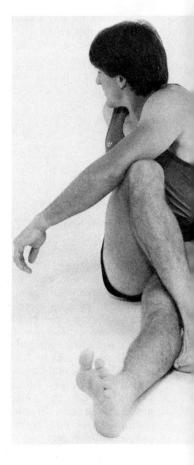

Sit on the floor with spine straight and legs outstretched (right). Bend the right leg and place the right foot on the outside of the left knee. Take the left arm and put it outside the bent right knee. Then place your right hand as far behind you as possible and turn your head to the rear.

Your left arm against the knee will act as a lever to enhance this stretch.

To increase the stretch, turn farther to the rear each time. Pause after each repetition and exhale. Do six repetitions, then switch and do six with the other leg. This means keeping the right leg straight, bending the left knee, and placing the left foot on the outside of the right knee. Then place the right arm on the outside of the left knee and turn as far as possible to the left and rear.

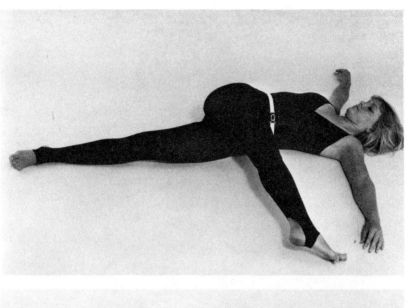

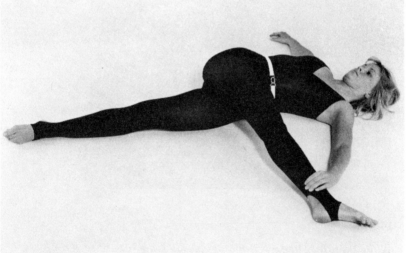

Lie flat on the floor with arms outstretched. Then raise the right leg and roll the leg over the body. Slowly move the leg farther to the left and up toward the head.

To increase the stretch, move the leg farther toward the head. Always keep both shoulders flat on the floor.

Pause after each repetition and exhale. Do six repetitions, then switch and do six with the other leg.

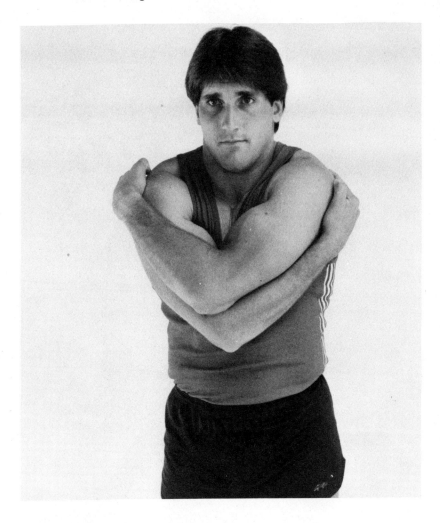

Upper Back

While this looks like a self-indulging "I like me" exercise, it really serves to stretch the upper back muscles (above).

Stand up straight and cross your arms across your chest, grasping as far back on the back as possible. One hand will be on top of the shoulder and the other under the arm.

Grip tightly with both hands. To increase the stretch, reach back even farther.

Pause after each repetition and exhale. Do six repetitions, then switch positions of hands and arms and do six more repetitions.

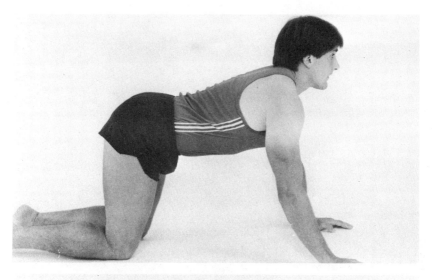

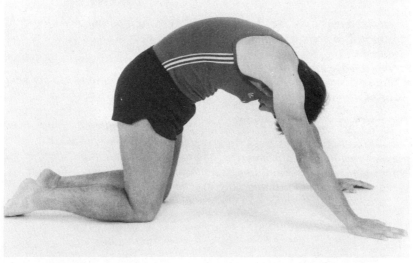

Lower Back

Kneel on all fours with legs close together and arms slightly farther apart than shoulder width. Back should be straight (above).

To do the stretch, arch the back as high as possible, as though reaching for the ceiling with the back.

To increase the stretch, reach even higher.

Pause after each repetition and exhale. Do six repetitions.

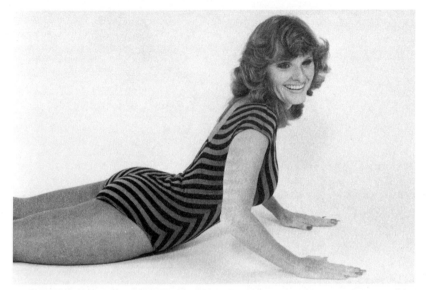

Lie flat on the floor, facedown (above). Keeping hips and pelvis touching the floor, do a press-up with the hands, raising your head and chest as high as possible.

To increase the stretch, raise higher each time.

Pause after each repetition and exhale. Do six repetitions. Always keep your hips and pelvis on the floor.

Below is a very relaxing way of stretching the overall body after a tense day. Lying flat on your back, keep your legs together and your arms at shoulder width. Attempt to reach with your hands as far as possible behind you, point your toes, and imagine that you are reaching with your feet toward an imaginary target. This, in essence, is a two-way stretch.

Pause after each repetition and exhale. Do six repetitions.

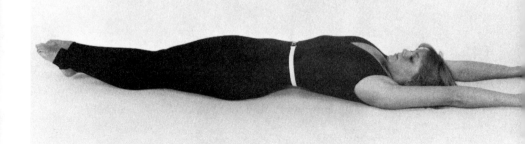

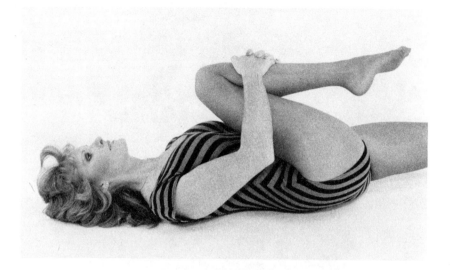

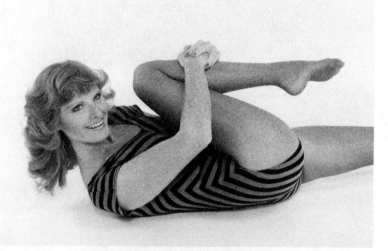

Lie flat on your back on the floor and keep your left leg outstretched. Raise your right knee to your chest. Attempt to touch the right knee to the right shoulder while holding the legs steady with arms wrapped over the upper part of the shin. Then move the leg so that it attempts to touch the left shoulder.

To increase the stretch, move the knee closer to the shoulder with each repetition.

Pause after each repetition and exhale. Do six repetitions, touching each shoulder each time; then switch and use the other leg.

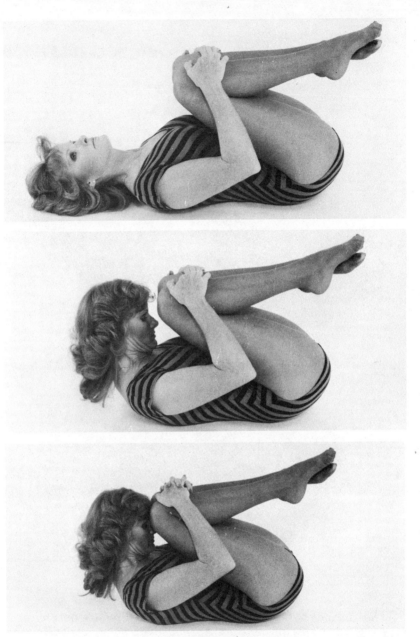

Lie flat on the floor on your back and bring both knees to the chest, grasping them with both hands wrapped around the upper part of the shins. Hold your knees as close as possible to your shoulders. Then raise your head in an attempt to touch the knees with your forehead.

This exercise almost becomes a rocking motion, as you increase the stretch by bringing the knees closer to the chest and your forehead closer to the knees, which can be done about 12 times.

Shoulders

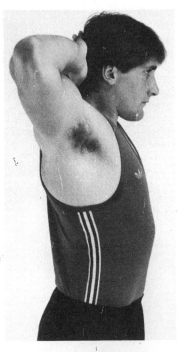

Stand up straight, then lace your fingers behind the head (left). Attempt to pull your elbows backward. To increase the stretch, pull the elbows farther back each time. Pause after each repetition and exhale. Do six repetitions.

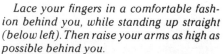

Lace your fingers in a comfortable fashion behind you, while standing up straight (below left). Then raise your arms as high as possible behind you.

To complete the full sequence, you will naturally bend from the waist as you go into further extension. To increase the stretch, reach higher each time. Pause after each repetition and exhale. Do six repetitions.

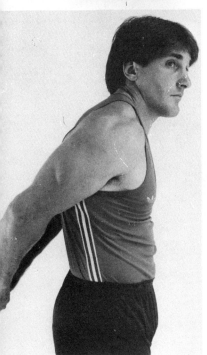

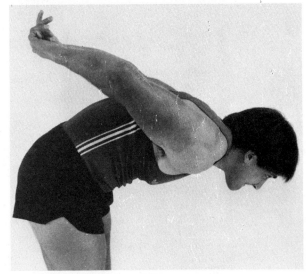

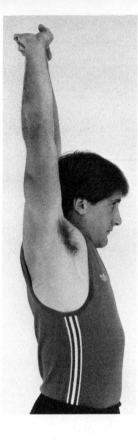
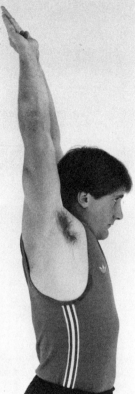

Interlock your thumbs and reach as high as possible while standing up straight (left). To increase the stretch, reach higher each time, with fingers pointing toward the ceiling. Pause after each repetition and exhale. Do six repetitions.

An alternative to this is to interlock the fingers with palms pointed upward and do six repetitions in this fashion. This slightly changes the area stretched in the shoulders.

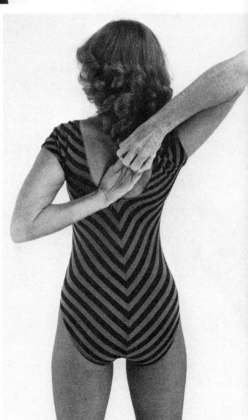

Reach behind you with the right arm over the top of the right shoulder and the left arm behind your back to try to grasp one hand with the other (right). To increase the stretch, clasp the hands together more tightly.

Most people can do this exercise in one direction, but when the hands are reversed so that the left hand is over the top of the left shoulder and the right hand comes up from behind, it is not as easy. A few people are able to do this easily in both directions. Pause after each repetition and exhale. Do six repetitions, then switch the position of both arms and repeat.

Neck

Neck stretches should be done slowly and carefully. The shoulders must remain in an upright level position.

Stand up straight, then attempt to touch the right ear to the right shoulder. The second variation is to touch the chin to the right shoulder. The third is to touch the chin to the chest, and the fourth is to touch the ear near the chest.

To increase these stretches, reach farther in the touching positions each time.

Pause after each repetition and exhale. Do six repetitions in each direction and in each touching position.

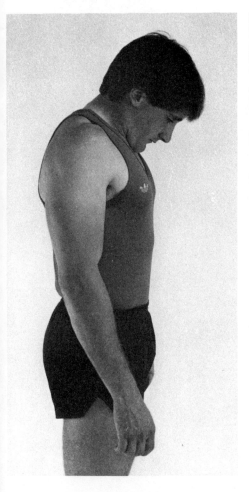 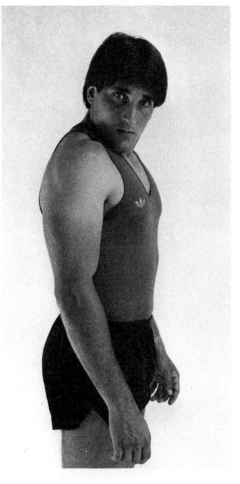

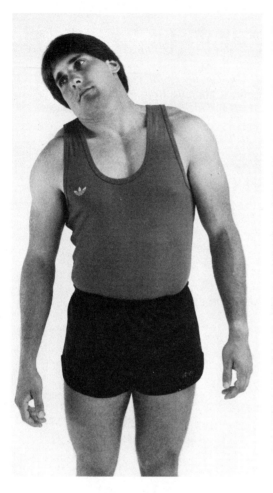
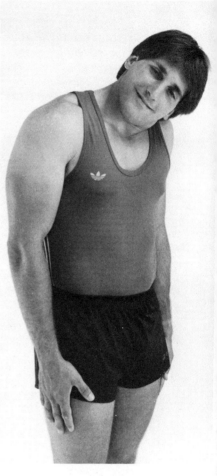

7

Hold-Relax Stretches

The Hold-Relax Technique

Hold-relax stretching is the safest and most productive of the three types of stretching. Studies have shown that after 10 minutes of static stretching you will achieve approximately a half-inch improvement in the range of motion. With proper hold-relax techniques you can obtain two to three inches of improvement in less time. So, whenever possible, incorporate hold-relax techniques into your routines.

Why is hold-relax superior? Hold-relax allows your body's own sensing mechanisms to aid in the stretching. First, by performing an isometric contraction, the body is supplying the muscle with blood; the contraction also creates a slight sense of fatigue in the muscle and it wants to relax when the contraction is stopped. Second, when one muscle is contracted, the opposite (or antagonistic) muscle is relaxed. For example, if you place a weight in your hand and bend your elbow, the brain sends out two signals. One signal instructs the bicep to contract; the other signal instructs the tricep to relax. Hold-relax uses this principle to relax the muscle it is stretching.

As soon as the isometric contraction is stopped, you contract the muscle on the opposite side of the joint. It is this message from the brain to the "stretched" muscle which actually causes the stretch to occur. The muscle that had been contracted isometrically relaxes, and its counterpart contracts, creating the stretch.

Hold-relax is actually very simple once you get the hang of it. Lie flat on your back on the floor with one leg out straight up in the air, perpendicular to the floor. The muscles that raise your leg in the air are called the hip flexors.

Now move the leg rapidly back toward the floor. The muscles that pulled your leg back to the starting point are the hamstrings. The hip flexors and the hamstrings are antagonist or opposite muscle groups.

Now raise the right leg in the air again. This time raise the leg until you feel a slight amount of tightness in the hamstrings. This is called *point of tightness* and means that, if you brought your legs back farther, you would feel pain. Reach up with both hands and grasp the right leg about the ankle. Now attempt to pull your leg back toward the floor using the hamstrings, while both hands hold the leg and prevent it from moving; this is called an *isometric contraction.* Continue to try to pull the leg toward the floor for five seconds. At the end of five seconds, stop contracting the hamstrings and immediately bring the leg back toward your head using the hip flexors. The leg will move back toward the head approximately one to two inches. This increase of one to two inches is called *increased range of motion.* You have now stretched the hamstring muscle using hold-relax. You should now do the same isometric contraction five more times, each time starting with the *new* range of motion.

Calf

Sit on the ground with one leg out straight and the other bent at the knee (page 63). Take the toes of the bent leg in both hands. Flex the toes to point toward the head.

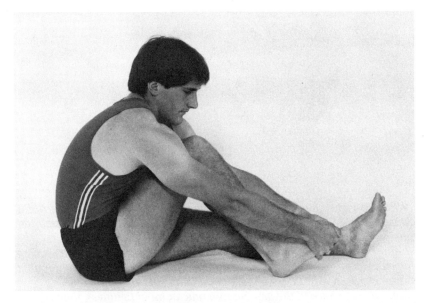

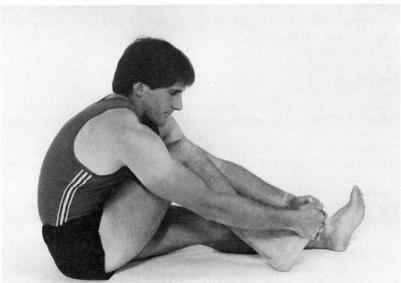

Using the calf muscle, push the toes toward the ground while slowly increasing the strength of the muscle contraction. Hands offer resistance.
Hold for five seconds, exhale, and relax.
Flex the toes more toward the head, then repeat the exercise.
Do six repetitions, then switch and use the other leg for six more.

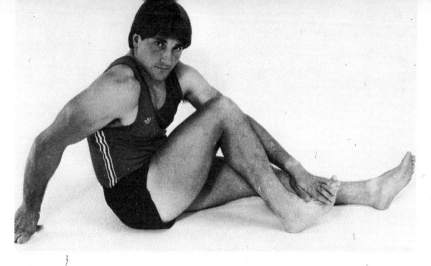

Shin

With the right knee bent and the left leg straight out on the ground (above), put the left hand on top of the right foot, which you have pointed out straight to a point of tightness.

Using the shin muscle, push the toes toward the head, slowly increasing the strength of the muscle contraction while the hands offer immovable resistance. Hold for five seconds, exhale, and relax.

Flex the toes toward the ground to a new point of tightness, then repeat the exercise.

Do six repetitions, then switch and do six with the other leg with the right hand on top of the left foot.

Hamstrings

Stretchers commonly perform this exercise (page 65) incorrectly, pulling their legs toward themselves without activating the hamstring and calf muscles.

Lie flat on the floor, keeping one leg outstretched at all times. Raise the other leg high to a point of tightness back toward your head, keeping the knees straight. Securely grasp the ankle or calf, whichever is more comfortable. Using the hamstring muscle, the large muscle on the underside of the upper part of your leg, attempt to push the leg back toward the ground while the hands offer an immovable resistance.

Slowly build the contraction of the muscle each time.

Hold for five seconds, exhale, and relax. Then move the leg closer to the head to a new point of tightness before repeating the exercise. Have the leg muscles move the leg back toward the head before repeating the exercise. Your hands are there to give the leg something to work against rather than just to "pull" the leg into a stretched position. Flex the toes so they try to point down toward the head on the final repetition. This enhances the stretch. Do six repetitions; then switch to the other leg for six more.

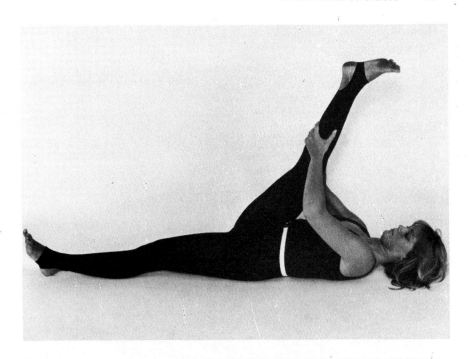

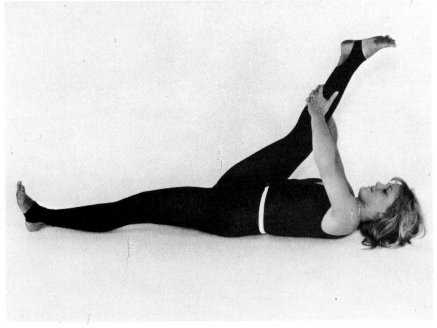

Thighs
(Quadriceps)

Lie facedown flat on the floor and grasp an ankle with one hand behind you. Tighten the thigh muscle. Using that muscle, attempt to straighten the leg back toward the ground, slowly building the strength of the muscle contraction while your hand offers immovable resistance. Hold for five seconds, exhale, and relax.

Using the hamstring muscle, pull your heel back toward the buttocks to a new point of tightness, then repeat the exercise. Do six repetitions, then switch to the other leg for six more.

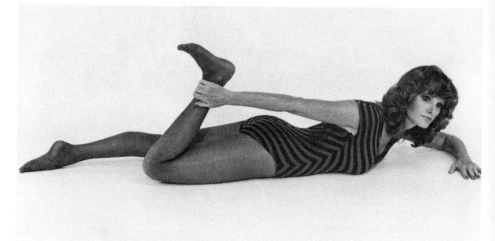

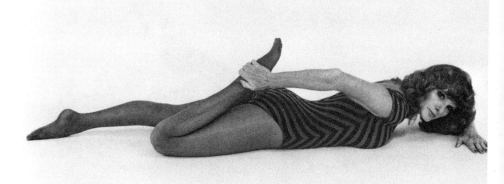

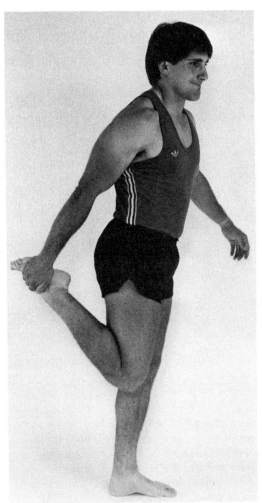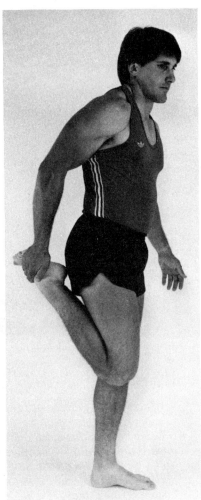

Standing up, raise one leg as high as possible behind you to a point of tightness, bending the knee. Grasp the foot or ankle.

Using the thigh muscle, push the foot toward the ground while slowly increasing the strength of muscle contraction. Your hand offers immovable resistance.

Hold for five seconds, exhale, and relax.

Using the hamstring muscle, bend your leg even farther to a new point of tightness, then repeat the exercise. Do six repetitions, then switch to the other leg for six more.

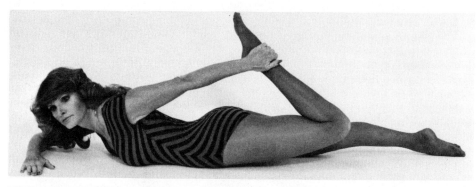

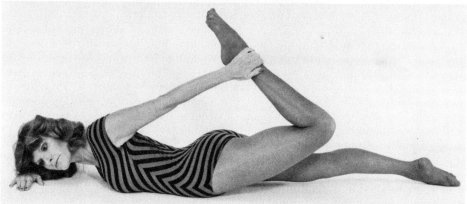

Hip Flexors

While lying facedown on the ground (above), lift the thigh off the ground to a point of tightness and grasp the ankle with the left hand.

Using the muscles in the front part of the hip, try to pull your knee back toward the ground, slowly increasing the strength of the muscle contraction. The left hand on the ankle offers immovable resistance.

Hold for five seconds, exhale, and relax. Raise the thigh and knee farther off the ground to a new point of tightness, then repeat the exercise.

Do six repetitions, then switch to the other leg for six more.

While lying on your side (page 69), raise your thigh and move the knee backward to a point of tightness; grasp the ankle with the left hand.

Using the muscles along the front part of the hip, try to pull your knee and toes forward, slowly increasing the strength of the muscle contraction.

Your hand on your ankle will offer immovable resistance.

Hold for five seconds, exhale, and relax.

Raise the leg higher and farther behind you to a new point of tightness, then repeat the exercise.

Do six repetitions, then switch to the other leg for six more.

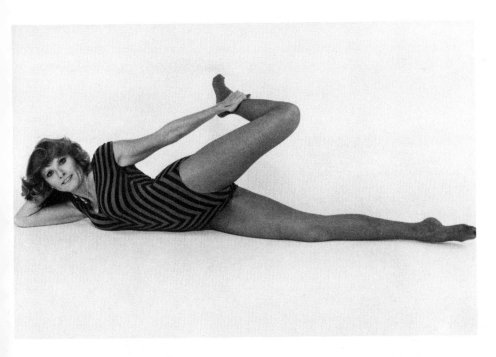

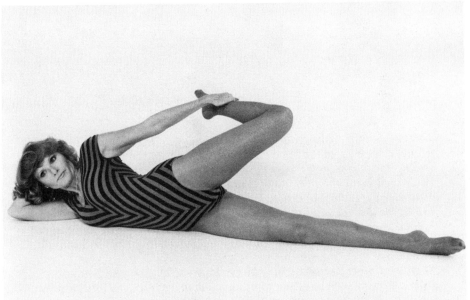

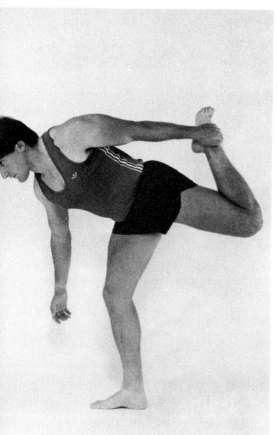 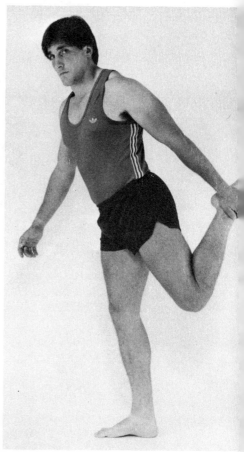

While standing with good posture, raise your left leg to a point of tightness, bending at the knee. Grasp the ankle with the left hand.

Using the hip muscles, pull the knee and foot directly forward while slowly increasing the strength of the muscle contraction. The hand on the ankle offers immovable resistance.

Hold for five seconds, exhale, and relax.

Move knee and foot farther backward to a new point of tightness, then repeat the exercise. Do six repetitions, then switch to the other leg for six more.

For less limber persons, it may be necessary to wrap a towel around the ankle and hold both ends of it to accomplish this exercise. It is natural for the upper body to lean forward while doing this exercise.

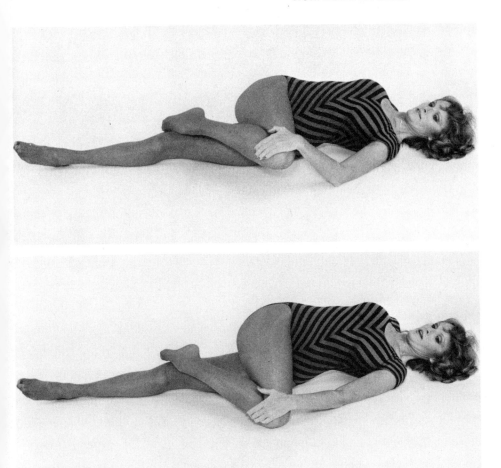

Sides
(Obliques)

Lie on your back, keeping both shoulders flat on the ground. Bend your right knee and roll it over the left outstretched leg toward the ground to a point of tightness. Put your left hand on top of the knee.

Using the side and hip muscles, push the right leg up while increasing the strength of the muscle contraction. The left hand offers immovable resistance. Hold for five seconds, exhale, and relax.

Using the side and hip muscles, move the bent leg more toward the ground to a new point of tightness, then repeat the exercise.

Do six repetitions, then switch to the other leg for six more.

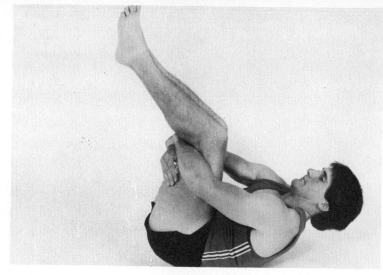

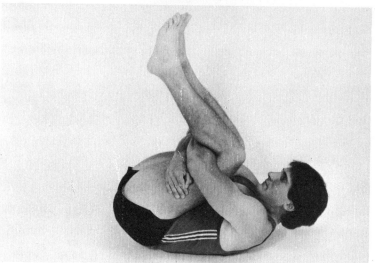

Lower Back

With your back flat on the floor, bring both knees to the chest to a point of tightness and wrap the arms around the upper legs. The more limber person will be able to wrap the arms around the entire bent leg with the hands going over the shins.

Using the lower back muscles, try to force the leg to break the immovable grasp provided by the hands as you increase the strength of the muscle contraction.

Hold for five seconds, exhale, and relax.

Pull the knees closer to the chest to a new point of tightness, then repeat the exercise.

Do six repetitions, then switch to the other leg for six more.

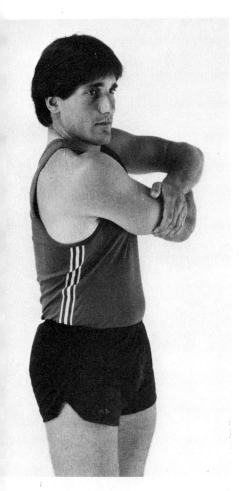 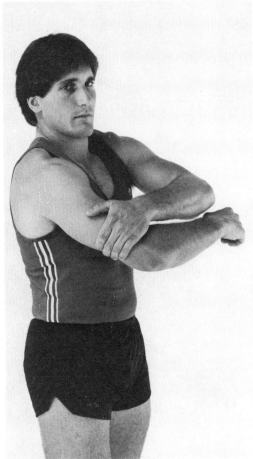

Upper Back

While standing up straight, hold the upper part of the right arm with the left hand, moving the arm to a point of tightness.

Using the muscles in the upper part of the back, slowly increase the strength of those contractions and attempt to hold the right arm away from the left hand, which is offering immovable resistance.

Hold for five seconds, exhale, and relax.

Move the right arm farther toward the left side to a new point of tightness, then repeat the exercise.

Do six repetitions, then switch to the other arm for six to be able to stretch the upper back muscles.

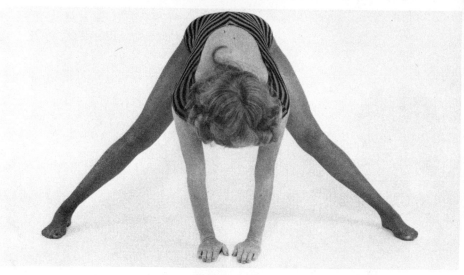

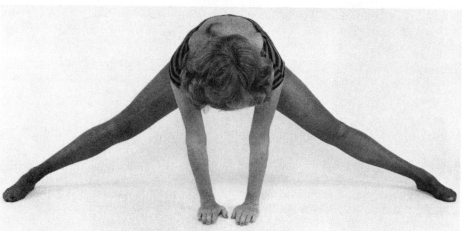

Groin

While standing, extend your legs as far apart as is comfortable and put your hands flat on the floor in front of you. Open the legs to a point of tightness.

Squeeze your feet into the floor. Slowly increase the strength of the muscle contraction of both the left and right groin while the ground is the immovable object.

Hold for five seconds, exhale, and relax.

Move the feet slightly farther apart to a new point of tightness, then repeat the exercise.

Do six repetitions.

It is vital to have a good grip on the floor with both feet, so be careful not to do this on a slick surface.

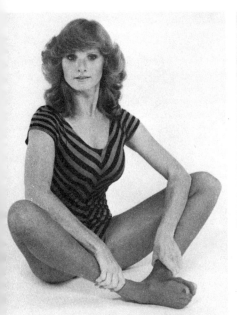 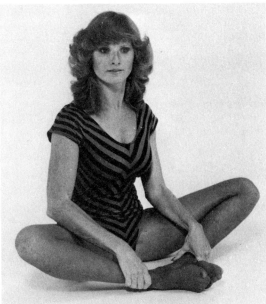

Sit upright on the ground, then pull the soles of your feet together as far as your legs can go back toward your body. Open your knees to a point of tightness. Grasp your feet with your hands so that your elbows rest on the inside of the knees.

Using the groin muscles, push your knees together, slowly increasing the strength of the muscle contraction with your elbows offering an immovable resistance.

Hold for five seconds, exhale, and relax.

Lower the knees more toward the floor to a new point of tightness, then repeat the exercise. It may also be possible to pull the feet a little closer to the body.

Do six repetitions.

Get into a squatting position with arms at shoulder width and balance on toes and fingertips (next page). Heels should be touching with knees apart at a point of tightness.

Using the groin muscles, slowly increase the strength of the muscle contraction while using the arms to offer immovable resistance to the inside of the legs.

Hold for five seconds, exhale, and relax.

Widen the position of the legs so that the knees are farther apart to a new point of tightness, then repeat the exercise.

Do six repetitions.

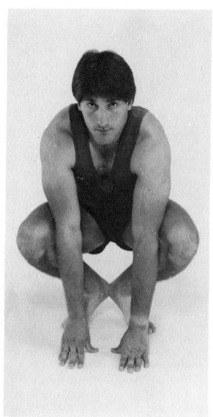
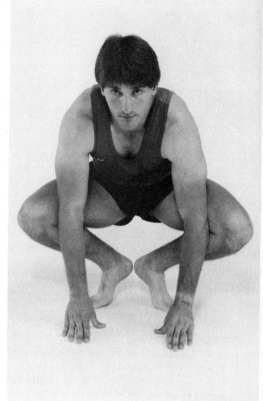

Shoulder

Stand up straight, raise the right arm above your head, and bend the elbow to a point of tightness (top of page 77). Elbow should be pointing straight ahead. Grasp the elbow with the left hand.

Using the upper back (latissimus dorsi) muscles, pull the elbow toward the ground, while slowly increasing the strength of the muscle contraction. The left hand provides immovable resistance to the exercise.

Hold for five seconds, exhale, and relax.

Move the arm farther toward the rear to a new point of tightness, then repeat the exercise.

Do six repetitions, then switch to the other arm for six more.

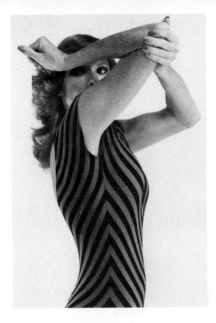 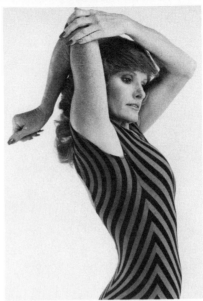

Neck

Standing up, tilt the chin toward the chest to a point of tightness and interlock fingers behind the head.

Using the neck muscles, push the back of the head against the hands, which offer an immovable resistance. Slowly increase the strength of the muscle contraction.

Hold for five seconds, exhale, and relax.

Move the chin closer to the chest to a new point of tightness, then repeat the exercise.

Do six repetitions.

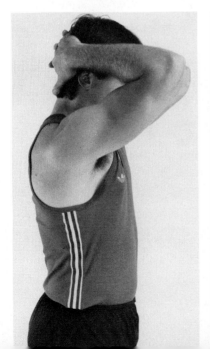 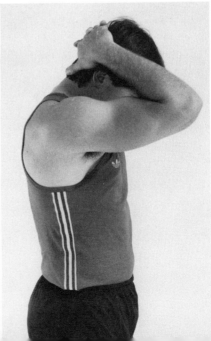

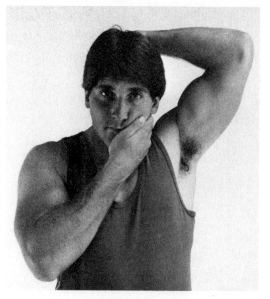 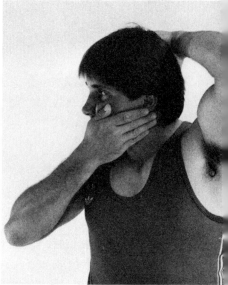

Standing up straight, place the left arm behind the head and the right hand against the side of the chin. Turn the head as far as possible to the right to a point of tightness.

Attempt to turn back to the left. Using the neck muscles, slowly increase the strength of the muscle contraction and push against the right hand with the chin. Your hand is an immovable resistance.

Hold for five seconds, exhale, and relax.

Turn the head farther to the right to a new point of tightness, then repeat the exercise.

Do six repetitions, then switch hands to the other side of the neck for six more.

8

Two-Person Stretches

Being stretched with a qualified person assisting you generally increases the intensity of the work and speeds flexibility growth. It also allows you to do some stretches your body usually can't do by itself because of limited range of motion.

The partner (coach, trainer, physical therapist) can urge you to work harder than you might otherwise by yourself. And the trained partner can feel when you are moving into new ranges of motion. But it has to be your responsibility to listen to your own body and not allow the stretcher to force you too far, thus tearing a muscle or straining a ligament or tendon.

Never try to work beyond your range. Straining in pain doesn't pay, despite clichés that suggest the opposite.

It's your body you are trying to improve, not the partner's. Pay attention to it.

If your part in a stretching routine is being the partner, remember you are there to give encouragement and to offer resistance, *not* to push or pull the other person into a new range.

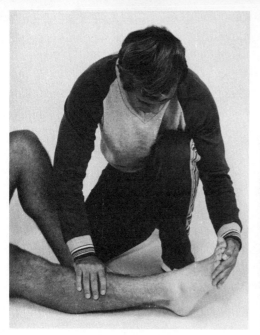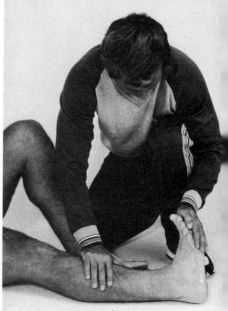

Calf and Achilles Tendon

Sit on the floor with left leg bent and the right leg outstretched.
The partner places one hand on the upper shin near the knee and the other hand on the sole of the right foot.
Flexed toes are pointed toward the head to the point of tightness.
Using the calf muscles, attempt to push the toes slowly toward the ground while increasing the strength of the muscle contraction.
Partner's hand provides immovable resistance.
Hold for five seconds, exhale, and relax.
Flex the toes more toward the head to a new point of tightness, then repeat the exercise.
Do six repetitions, then switch to the other leg for six more.

Shin

Sit flat on the floor with right leg outstretched and left leg bent (top of page 81). Point the right toes to a point of tightness, then have your partner hold the leg with one hand near the knee and the other hand resting on the top of the toes.
Using the shin muscles, attempt to pull the toes toward your head while slowly increasing the strength of the muscle contraction, while your partner's hand provides immovable resistance.
Hold for five seconds, exhale, and relax.
Point the toes farther toward the ground to a new point of tightness, then repeat the exercise.
Do six repetitions, then switch to the other leg for six more.

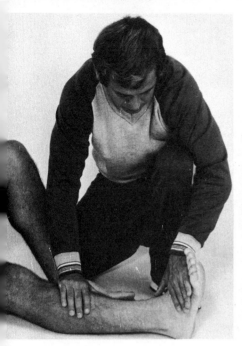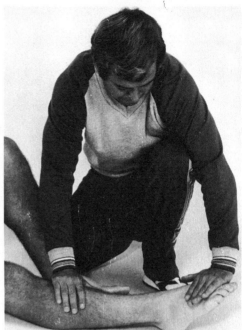

Hamstrings

Lie flat on the floor, then raise the left leg to a point of tightness without bending the knee. Partner will brace his shoulder against your calf while holding your right knee with the left hand to keep the right leg from coming off the floor (below).

Using the hamstring muscle, attempt to push the foot back toward the floor while slowly increasing the strength of the muscle contraction (top of page 82). Partner's shoulder provides immovable resistance.

Hold for five seconds, exhale, and relax.

Move the left leg farther toward the head to a new point of tightness, then repeat the exercise.

Do six repetitions, then switch to the other leg for six more.

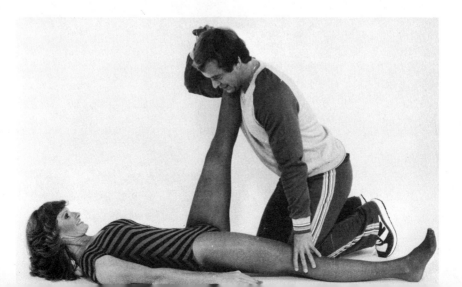

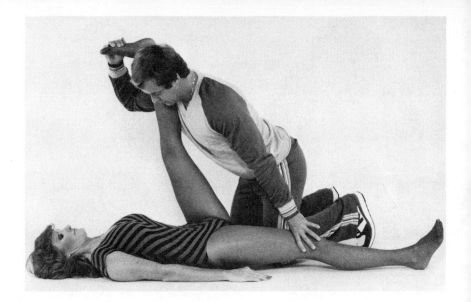

Lie flat on the floor, keeping the right leg straight. Raise the left leg, bending it so that the knee can touch the chest (below).

Hold your hamstring muscle with both hands. The partner then will brace with one hand over your hand and the other against your left heel.

Contract the hamstring muscle, pulling your heel into the partner's palm.

Using the thigh muscle, push the heel back toward the ground, while slowly increasing the strength of the muscle contraction (top of page 83). Partner's hand offers immovable resistance to the heel.

Hold for five seconds, exhale, and relax.

Rebend the knee, pulling it closer to the chest, then straighten the leg to a new point of tightness before repeating the exercise.

Do six repetitions, then switch to the other leg for six more.

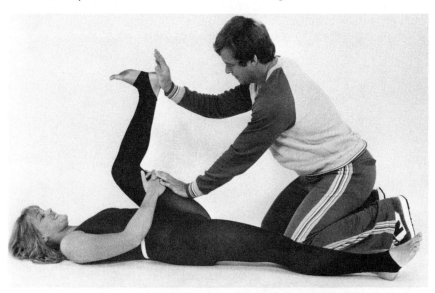

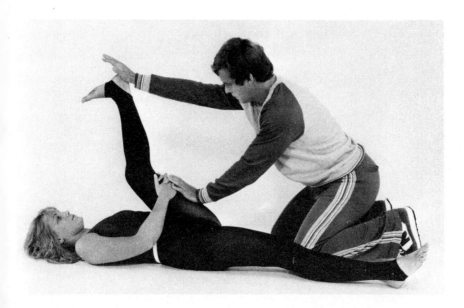

Thighs
(Quadriceps)

Lie facedown on the floor, then bend the right knee to a point of tightness. Partner will grasp the right ankle with both hands (below).

Using the thigh muscle, push the toes back toward the ground while slowly increasing strength of the muscle contraction (top of page 84). Partner's hands will offer immovable resistance.

Hold for five seconds, exhale, and relax.

Bend the knee even farther to a new point of tightness, then repeat the exercise.

Do six repetitions, then switch to the other leg for six more.

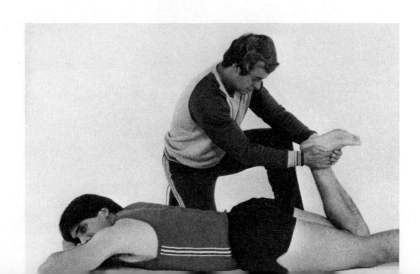

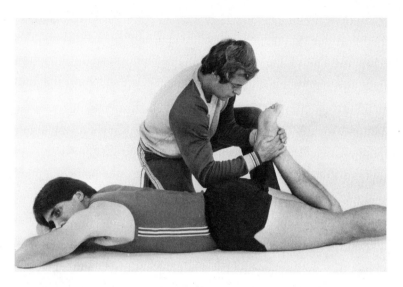

Hip Flexors

Lie facedown on the floor, with left leg outstretched. Bend the right leg as much as possible, then raise the right knee off the ground to a point of tightness. Partner places one hand in the small of your back, and the other holding the right knee (below).

Using the hip muscles, attempt to drive the knee back toward the ground, while slowly increasing the strength of the muscle contraction (top of page 85). Partner's hand on the knee provides immovable resistance.

Hold for five seconds, exhale, and relax.

Raise the knee even higher to a new point of tightness, then repeat the exercise.

Do six repetitions, then switch to the other leg for six more.

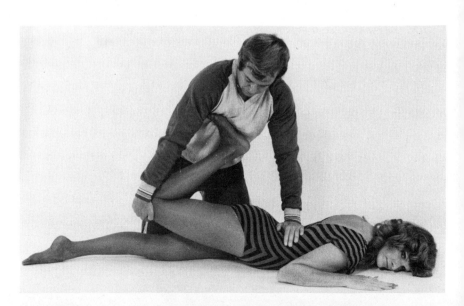

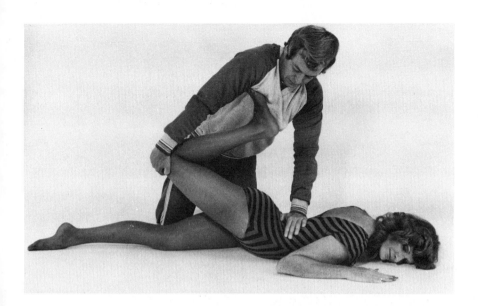

Groin

Sit up straight, then bend your knees and pull your feet together, with your heels touching, to a point of tightness. Brace yourself with both hands outspread and slightly behind you. Partner puts his hands on the inside of each knee (below).

Using your groin muscles, attempt to push the knees upward while slowly increasing the strength of the muscle contraction (top of page 86). Partner's hands provide immovable resistance.

Hold for five seconds, exhale, and relax.

Move your knees closer to the ground and pull the heels slightly closer to your body to a new point of tightness, then repeat the exercise.

Do six repetitions, then switch to the other leg for six more.

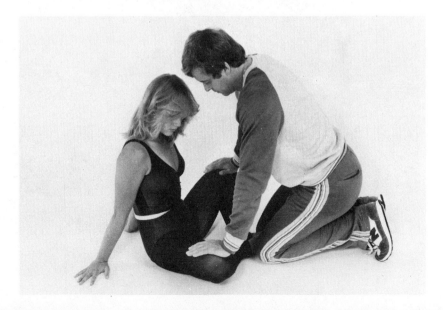

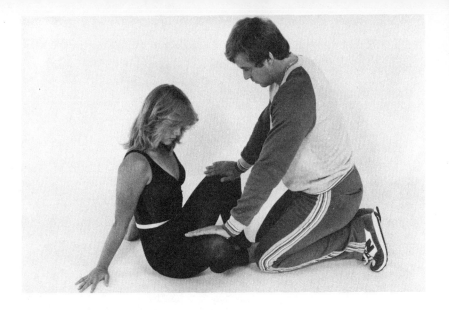

Lower Back

Sit with legs spread as far apart as is comfortable, then reach forward to a new point of tightness. Partner places both hands on the upper back (below).

Using the lower back muscles, push the back toward an upright sitting position, while slowly increasing the strength of the muscle contraction (top of page 87). Partner's hands provide immovable resistance.

Hold for five seconds, exhale, and relax.

Reach farther forward to a new point of tightness, then repeat the exercise. Do six repetitions.

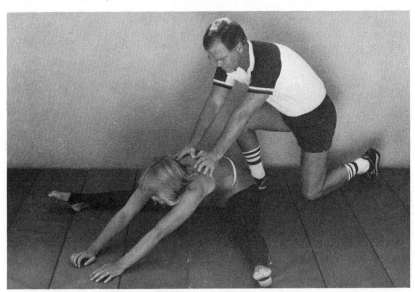

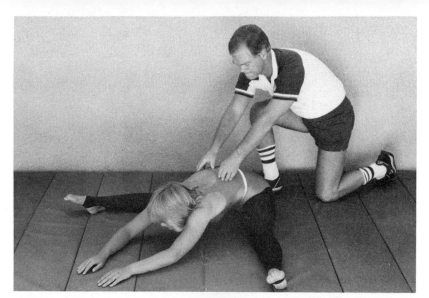

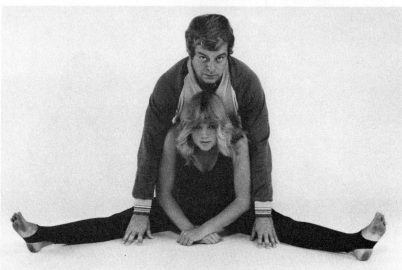

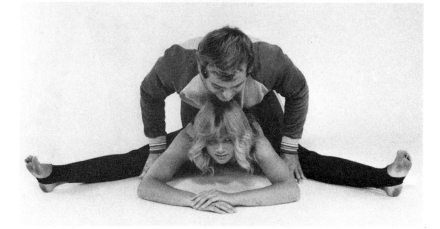

Hip Flexors and Quadriceps

Stand upright and lean forward slightly, bracing against a wall or another solid object. Raise your left leg, bending it, to a point of tightness.

Partner puts one hand against the small of your back and the other grasps the ankle.

Using the hip muscles, attempt to push your foot back toward the ground against the immovable resistance of the partner's hand on the ankle, while slowly increasing the strength of the muscle contraction.

Hold for five seconds, exhale, and relax.

Bend your knee even farther to a new point of tightness, then repeat the exercise.

Do six repetitions, then switch to the other side for six more.

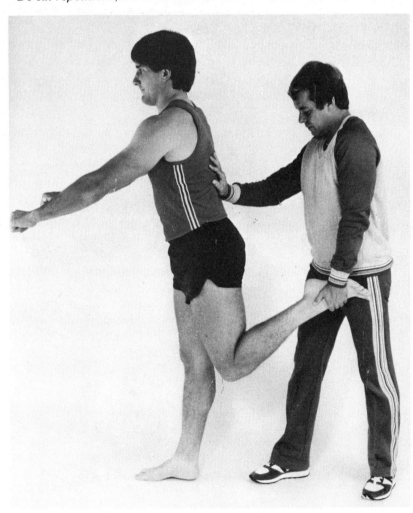

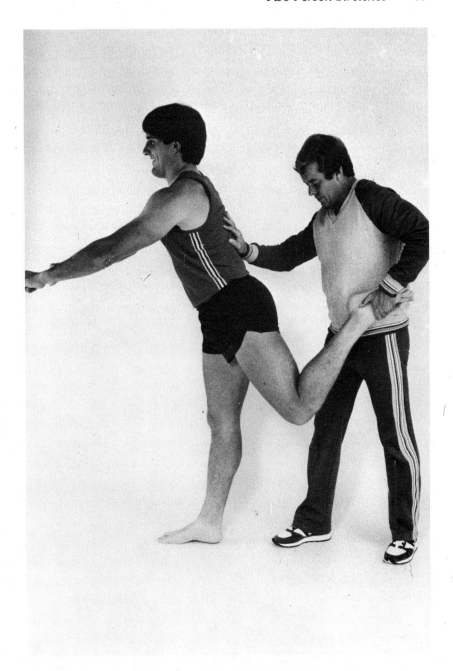

Lower Back

Sit upright with legs outstretched and together. Reach forward to a point of tightness. Partner places his chest against your upper back.

Using your back muscles, push upward while slowly increasing the strength of the muscle contraction. Partner's chest provides immovable resistance.

Hold for five seconds, exhale, and relax.

Reach farther forward to a new point of tightness, then repeat the exercise.

Do six repetitions.

Partner must not push on your back to create a new range of motion. You must control the exercise.

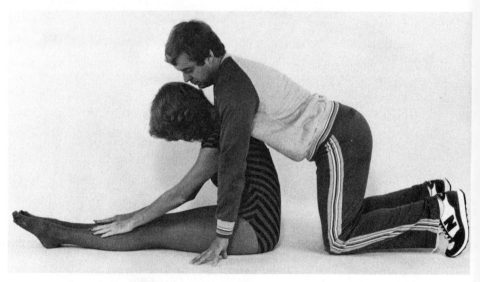

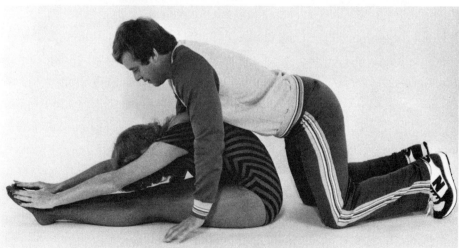

Hamstrings and Groin

This exercise primarily stretches the hamstrings, but works on the groin area as well.

Sit with legs spread as far apart as is comfortable, then reach toward the right foot to a point of tightness. Partner places his hands on your upper back.

Using the lower back muscles, push backward while slowly increasing the strength of the muscle contraction. Partner's hands offer an immovable resistance.

Hold for five seconds, exhale, and relax.

Reach farther toward the right foot to a new point of tightness, then repeat the exercise.

Do six repetitions, then switch to the other leg for six more.

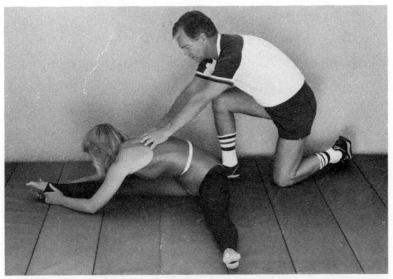

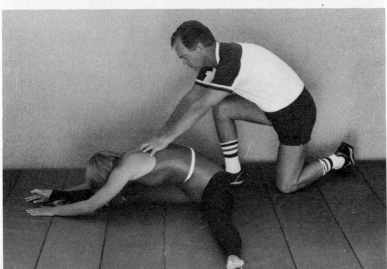

Side Stretches
(Obliques)

Sit upright on the ground with legs outstretched and knees apart. Turn to the left to a point of tightness. Partner places hands at the points of each shoulder. Look straight ahead.

Using the side (oblique) muscles, try to turn to the right, slowly increasing the strength of the muscle contraction.

For maximum resistance, partner shouldn't bend forward at the waist. Hold for five seconds, exhale, and relax.

Turn back to the left to a new point of tightness, then repeat the exercise, attempting to turn farther to the left.

Do six repetitions, then switch and turn the other way for six more.

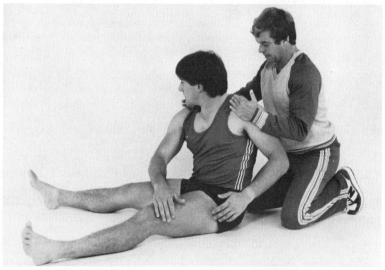

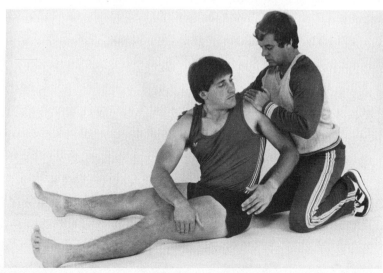

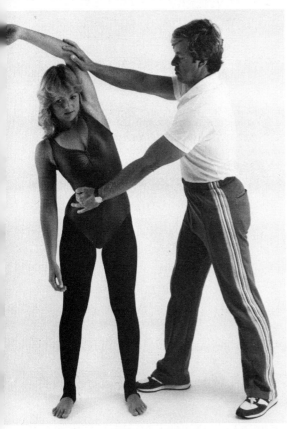

Stand upright with feet spread apart at shoulder width. Raise the left arm as high as possible and bend to the right. Reach with the right hand toward the right knee to a point of tightness. Partner places one hand around your waist and the other against your left elbow.

Using the left side muscles, attempt to straighten up against the immovable resistance of your partner's hands while slowly increasing the strength of the muscle contraction. Hold for five seconds, exhale, and relax.

Reach farther down the right leg to a new point of tightness, then repeat the exercise. Do six repetitions, then switch to the other side for six more. Be certain not to bend forward at the waist while performing the exercise. Bend directly to the side.

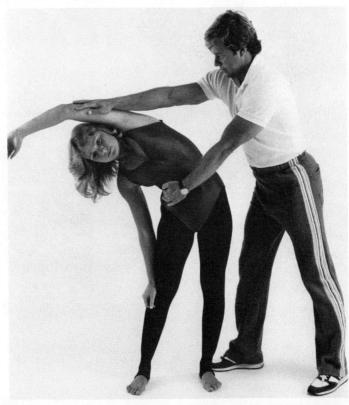

Shoulders

Sit on the floor with legs outstretched and arms raised directly over-head. Partner kneels behind with knees against your buttocks and lightly grasps your wrists. Reach back to a point of tightness.

Using the chest and upper back (latissimus dorsi) muscles, push your arms forward toward the ground, while slowly increasing the strength of the muscle contraction. Note that partner doesn't pull arms back; he just provides resistance.

Hold for five seconds, exhale, and relax.

Reach farther backward to a new point of tightness, then repeat the exercise.

Do six repetitions.

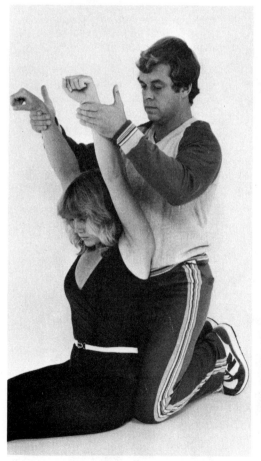 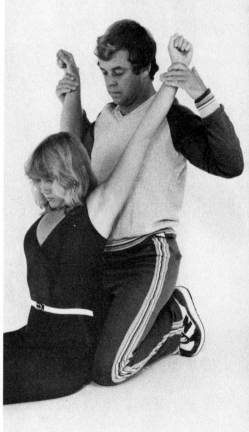

Sit up straight on the ground or in a chair and interlock your fingers behind your head with your elbows pointed out. Partner braces against your back and lightly grasps the inside of each elbow.

Bend your arms as far backward as possible, then contract the chest muscles (pectorals).

Using the chest muscles, attempt to pull your elbows forward, while slowly increasing the strength of the muscle contraction. Partner's hands offer immovable resistance.

Hold for five seconds, exhale, and relax.

Move elbows farther backward to a new point of tightness, then repeat the exercise.

Do six repetitions.

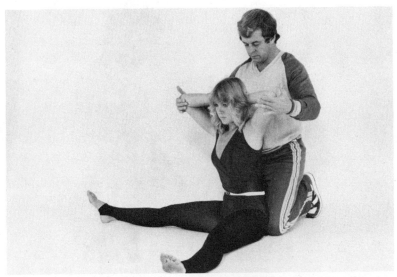

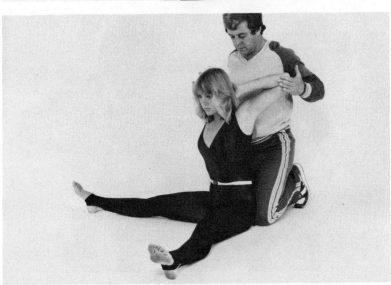

Shoulders

Stand up straight and move both arms backwards to a point of tightness as far as possible. Partner grasps each wrist lightly.

Using your shoulder muscles, pull the arms forward, slowly increasing the strength of the muscle contractions in the shoulders. Partner's hands offer immovable resistance.

Hold for five seconds, exhale, and relax.

Extend the arms farther backward to a new point of tightness, then repeat the exercise.

Do six repetitions.

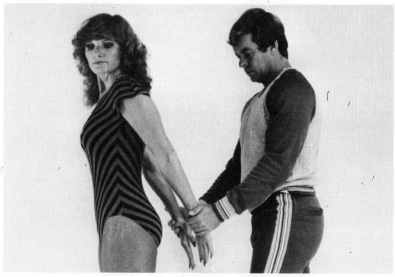

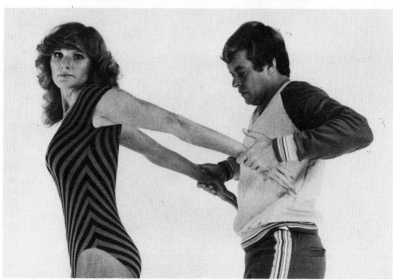

Shoulder Rotation

This exercise is particularly good for warming up pitchers, quarterbacks, javelin throwers.

Stand upright and place your arm in a position as though you were going to throw a ball overhand. The arm is bent at the elbow at a 90-degree angle with the hand above the head and back at a point of tightness. Partner places one hand on your inner elbow and the other on your hand.

Using the shoulder muscles, slowly move the hand toward the front as though you were throwing a ball, while slowly increasing the strength of the muscle contractions. Partner's hand offers immovable resistance.

Hold for five seconds, exhale, and relax.

Move the hand farther to the rear to a new point of tightness, then repeat the exercise.

Do six repetitions, then switch to the other arm for six more.

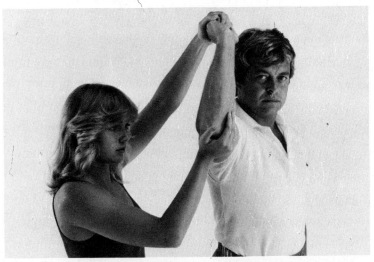

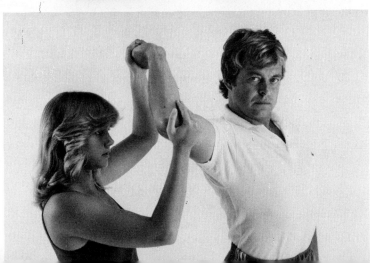

Tricep

Standing up straight, extend your arm out, then bend the elbow so that the hand is facing the ground and bent backward to a point of tightness. Partner places one hand against the inside of the elbow and holds the top part of your hand with his hand.

Rotate the shoulder backward.

Using the tricep muscles, attempt to move your hand forward while slowly increasing the strength of the muscle contraction. Partner's hand offers immovable resistance.

Hold for five seconds, exhale, and relax.

Bend the elbow farther to the back to a new point of tightness, then repeat the exercise.

Do six repetitions, then switch to the other arm for six more.

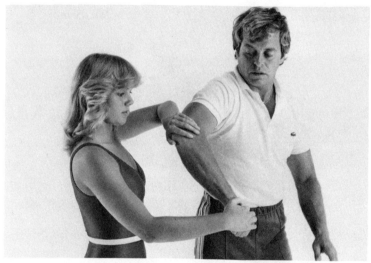

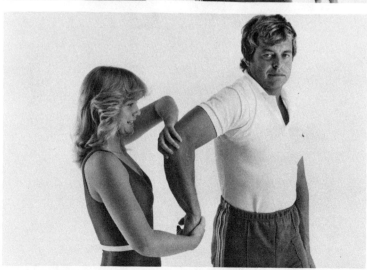

Upper Back
(Latissimus Dorsi)

Stand up straight and cross your arms across your chest to a point of tightness with the hands pointing in opposite directions. Partner places a hand on the upper arm side of each elbow.

Using the back (latissimus dorsi) muscles, attempt to uncross your arms while slowly increasing the strength of the muscle contraction. Partner's hands offer immovable resistance to your elbow movement. Hold for five seconds, exhale, and relax.

Move hands farther to the rear to a new point of tightness, then repeat the exercise.

Do six repetitions.

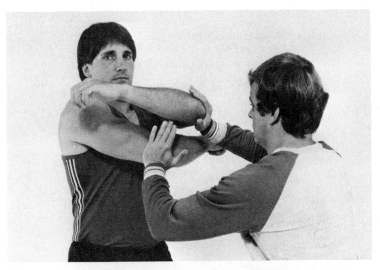

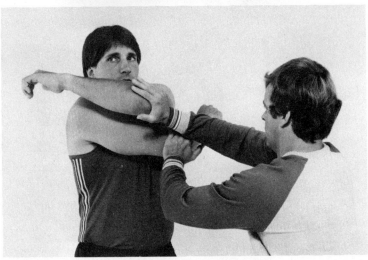

Upper Back
(Latissimus Dorsi)

Stand up straight and raise one hand above your head and bend at the elbow, reaching behind you to a point of tightness. Partner places one hand on your lower back and the other at your elbow.

Using the chest and upper back (latissimus dorsi) muscles, attempt to drive your arm forward toward the ground, while slowly increasing the strength of the muscle contraction. Partner's hand offers immovable resistance at the elbow.

Reach farther behind you with your hand to a new point of tightness, then repeat the exercise.

Do six repetitions, then switch to the other arm for six more.

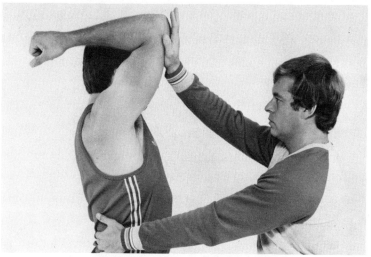

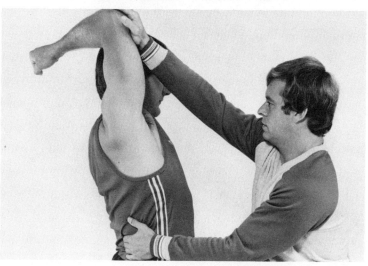

Lower Back

This is an excellent stretch for the lower back. Lie flat on the ground, keeping both shoulders in contact at all times. Leave your left leg stretched out straight, but bend the right leg at the knee to a point of tightness, then roll the knee over the left leg, attempting to touch it to the ground on the other side.

Partner places one hand on your right shoulder and the other on the outside of your right knee.

Using the muscles of your lower back, attempt to raise your knee while slowly increasing the strength of the muscle contraction. Partner's hand on your knee offers immovable resistance.

Hold for five seconds, exhale, and relax.

Bend your leg farther to a new point of tightness, then repeat the exercise.

Do six repetitions, then switch to the other leg for six more.

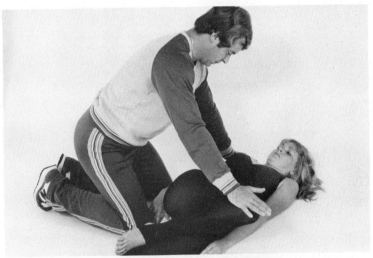

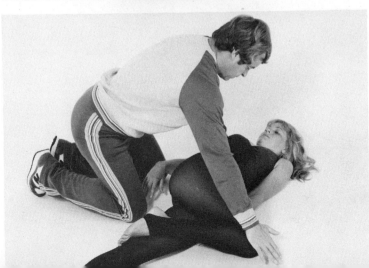

Lie flat on the floor, then pull both legs upward and bring your knees as close to your chest to a point of tightness. Partner kneels and places his chest against the soles of your feet, each of you grasping the other's arms.

Using the back muscles, push with your feet against the partner's chest while slowly increasing the strength of the muscle contraction. Partner's chest offers immovable resistance.

Hold for five seconds, exhale, and relax.

Bring your knees closer to your chest to a new point of tightness, then repeat the exercise.

Do six repetitions.

This is a pushing exercise, not a kicking maneuver.

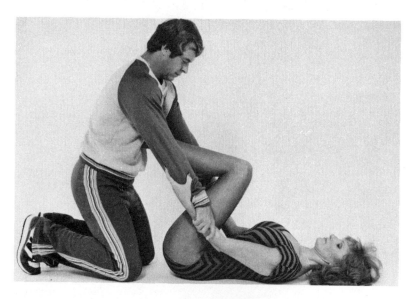

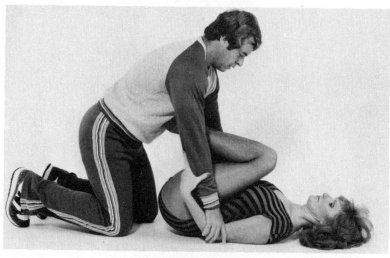

Neck

Sit upright, then have your partner place one hand behind your head as a brace and the other hand under your chin. Turn your head to a point of tightness to one side.

Using the neck muscles, turn your chin back toward the front, slowly increasing the strength of the muscle contraction. Partner's hand on the chin offers immovable resistance.

Hold for five seconds, exhale, and relax.

Turn the head farther to the side to a new point of tightness, then repeat the exercise.

Do six repetitions, then switch and turn the head the other way for six more.

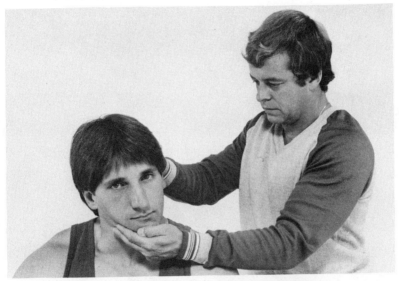

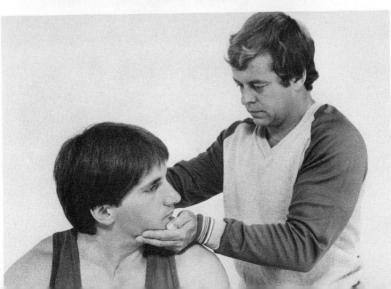

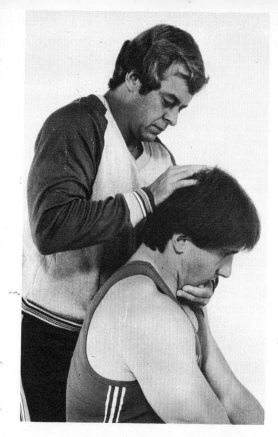

Sit upright and have your partner place one hand against the back of your head and the other under your chin. Tilt your head forward to a point of tightness.

Using the neck muscles, push backward with your head while slowly increasing the strength of the muscle contraction. Partner's hand on the back of your head offers immovable resistance. Hold for five seconds, exhale, and relax.

Bend your head farther forward to a new point of tightness, then repeat the exercise. Do six repetitions.

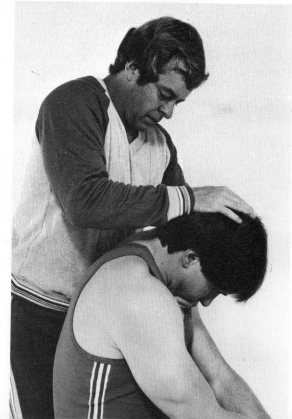

Upper Shoulders

Sit upright, then have partner place a hand on top of each shoulder. You will be attempting to raise your shoulders in this exercise, first lowering the shoulders to a point of tightness.

Using the shoulder muscles, push upward with both shoulders, while slowly increasing the strength of the muscle contraction. Partner's hands on your shoulders offer immovable resistance.

Hold for five seconds, exhale, and relax.

Lower the shoulders farther to a new point of tightness, then repeat the exercise.

Do six repetitions.

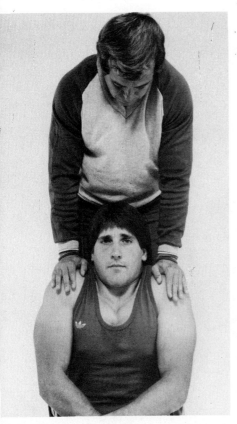 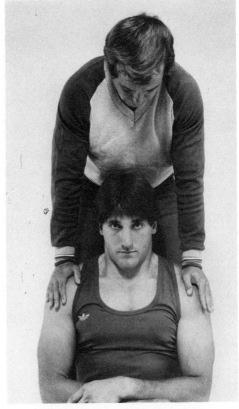

9

Apparatus Stretches

When you stretch by yourself, frequently there are some exercises in the beginning that you can't do. You might not be able to reach your ankle to do a proper Straight-Leg Hamstring Stretch or grasp the ankle from behind for Thigh and Hip Flexor Stretches.

A bath towel looped over the ankle allows you to work on stretches that you should be able to accomplish with your hands as you gain flexibility over time.

A cable or rope pulley apparatus with a handle on one end and a Velcro strap on the other also can speed up the process.

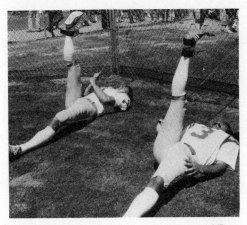

A rope pulley apparatus is ideal for athletes who wish to regulate their own training.

107

The apparatus will allow team members to do more stretching because each athlete can look after his own program. Several types of apparatus can be attached to a wall in the locker room or to hooks on a gymnasium wall or along a fence. This way, several players can stretch simultaneously.

TOWEL STRETCHES

Calf

Sit flat on the floor with both legs outstretched. Loop a towel over the right foot while the toes are pointed straight up to a point of tightness (below).

Using the calf muscle, push the toes toward the floor while slowly increasing the strength of the muscle contraction (page 109). The towel offers immovable resistance to the push.

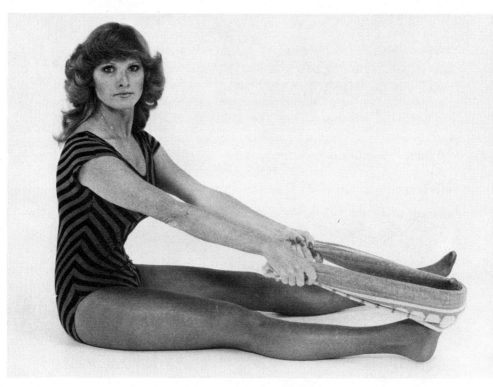

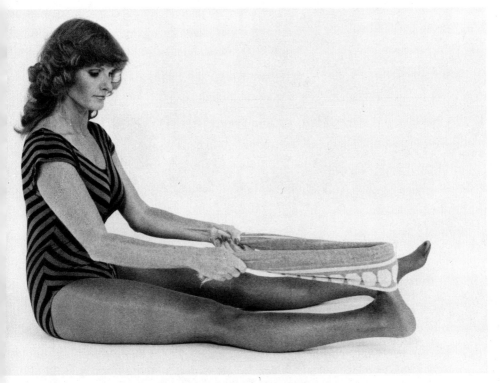

Hold for five seconds, exhale, and relax. Flex the toes farther toward the head to a new point of tightness, then repeat the exercise.

Do six repetitions, then switch to the other leg for six more.

Hamstrings

Lie flat on your back with the left leg outstretched and the right leg raised to a point of tightness while keeping the knee straight (see top of page 110). Loop a towel over the right heel.

Using the hamstring, push the leg toward the floor, slowly increasing the strength of the muscle contraction, while the towel offers immovable resistance.

Hold for five seconds, exhale, and relax. Move the leg farther back toward the head to a new point of tightness while keeping the knee straight. Repeat the exercise.

Do six repetitions, then switch to the left leg for six more.

Remember not to pull the leg with the towel. Allow the hip flexors to move the leg into a new range of motion.

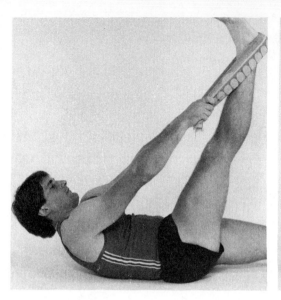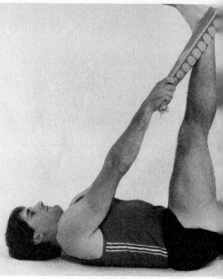

Thighs

While lying flat on your stomach, bend your left leg to a point of tightness toward your head.

Loop a towel around the ankle.

Using the thigh muscle, push your foot back toward the ground while slowly increasing the strength of the muscle contraction while the towel offers immovable resistance.

Hold for five seconds, exhale, and relax.

Bend the leg to a new point of tightness, then repeat the exercise.

Do six repetitions, then switch to the other leg for six more.

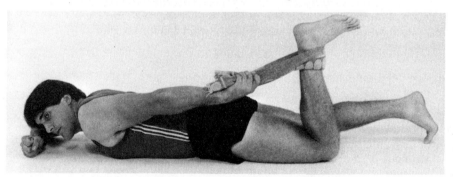

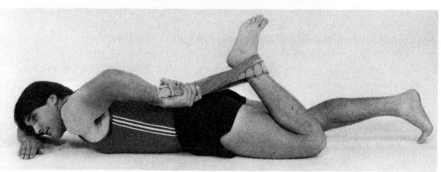

Hip Flexor

Lie facedown, flat on the floor, then bend the left leg toward the head to a point of tightness. Loop a towel around the left ankle and grasp it with the right hand. Raise your left leg off the ground to a point of tightness.

Using the hip flexor muscles, push the knee back toward the ground while slowly increasing the strength of the muscle contraction. The towel offers immovable resistance.

The movement of the leg is up and in at a 45-degree angle, as though you are trying to touch your left heel to your right shoulder.

Hold for five seconds, exhale, and relax.

Raise the leg even higher to a new point of tightness, then repeat the exercise.

Do six repetitions, then switch to the right leg, holding the towel with the left hand, for six more.

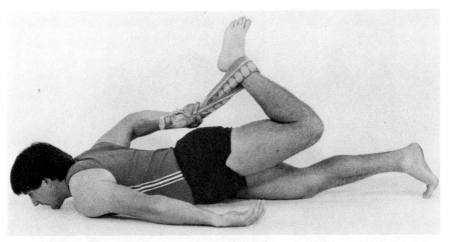

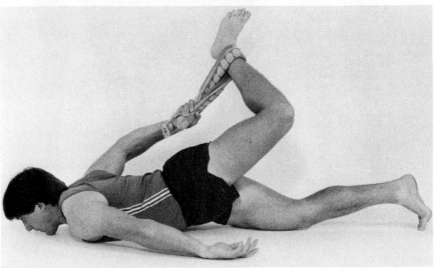

Sides
(Obliques)

Stand with both feet shoulder width apart, while anchoring one end of a long towel. Grasp the towel with the right hand to a point of tightness. Bend directly to the side, not forward at the waist.

Using the left side muscles, slowly increase the strength of the muscle contraction, pulling hard on the towel with the right hand, while the towel offers immovable resistance to the stretch.

Hold for five seconds, exhale, and relax.

Grasp the towel farther down toward the ground to a new point of tightness along the side, then repeat the exercise.

Do six repetitions, then switch to the other side for six more.

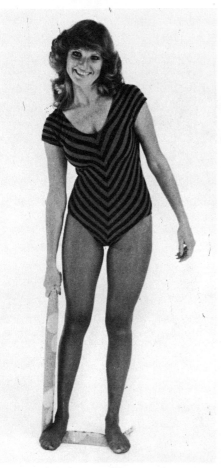 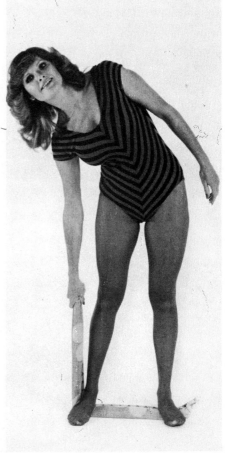

Upper Back

Wrap the towel across the broadest part of your shoulders and grip it with arms crossed to a point of tightness.

Using the upper back muscles, attempt to pull the towel ends closer together, slowly increasing the strength of the muscle contractions, while the towel offers immovable resistance.

Hold for five seconds, exhale, and relax. Move the hands farther toward the opposite shoulders to a new point of tightness, then repeat the exercise.

Do six repetitions.

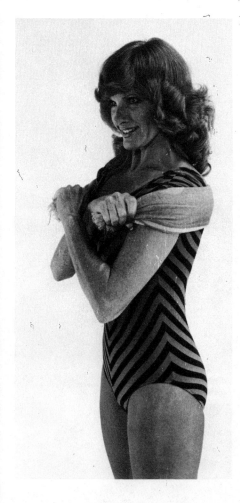 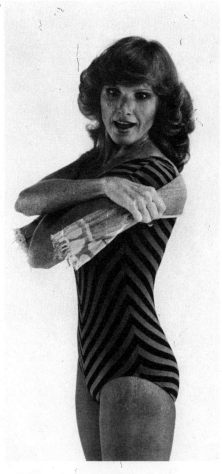

Lower Back

Lie flat on your back on the floor, then bring your knees to your chest to a point of tightness and loop a towel over the bottoms of both feet.

Using the lower back muscles, push upward with both feet, while slowly increasing the strength of the muscle contraction. The towel offers immovable resistance.

Hold for five seconds, exhale, and relax.

Regrip the towel while moving the knees even closer to the chest to a new point of tightness, then repeat the exercise.

Do six repetitions.

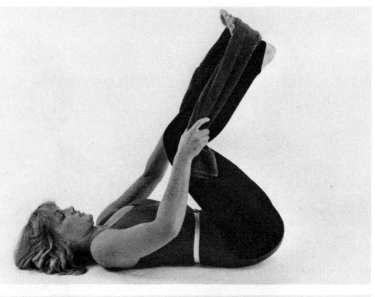

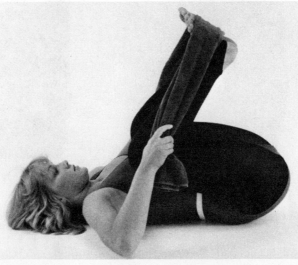

CABLE-PULLEY APPARATUS

Hamstrings

Attach the strap on the left ankle, then lie flat on the floor with your head pointing toward the pulley. Grasp the pulley handle with the left hand and raise the left leg to a point of tightness toward the head.

Using the hamstring muscle, push the leg back toward the ground while slowly increasing the strength of the muscle contraction. The hand holding the other end of the cable offers immovable resistance.

Hold for five seconds, exhale, and relax.

Raise the leg even higher toward the head to a new point of tightness, then repeat the exercise.

Do six repetitions, then switch to the other leg for six more.

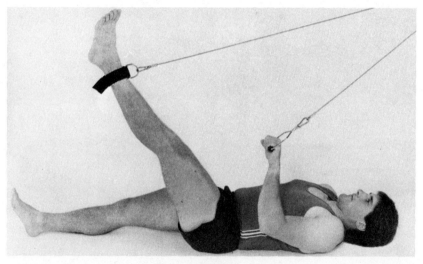

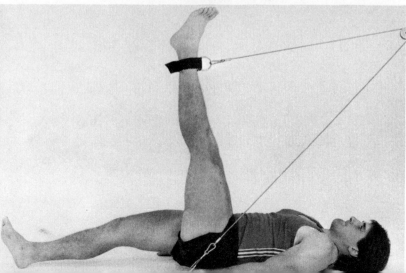

Attach the cable strap to the left ankle, then lie flat on the ground with the head toward the pulley apparatus and hold the other end of the cable with the left hand. Raise the left leg and attempt to touch the knee to the chest, then straighten the leg to a point of tightness.

Using the thigh muscle, try to drive the foot back toward the ground, slowly increasing the strength of the muscle contraction. The left hand holding the other end of the cable provides immovable resistance.

Hold for five seconds, exhale, and relax.

Move the knee closer to the head and straighten the leg out even farther to a new point of tightness, then repeat the exercise.

Do six repetitions, then switch to the other leg for six more.

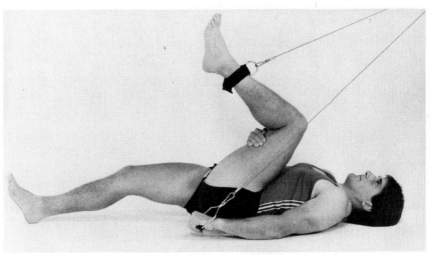

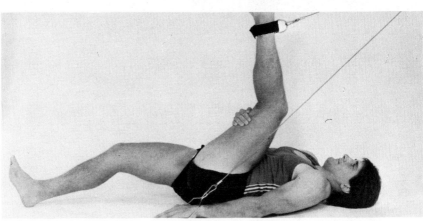

Thighs
(Quadriceps)

Attach the strap at one end of the cable to the right leg, then lie flat on the stomach, facing the pulley attachment. Bend the right knee to a point of tightness.

Using the thigh muscle, try to force the toes of your foot back toward the floor, while slowly increasing the strength of the muscle contraction and using the right hand holding the other end of the cable to offer immovable resistance.

Hold for five seconds, exhale, and relax.

Raise the leg even farther and bend the knee more to a new point of tightness, then repeat the exercise.

Do six repetitions, then switch to the other leg for six more.

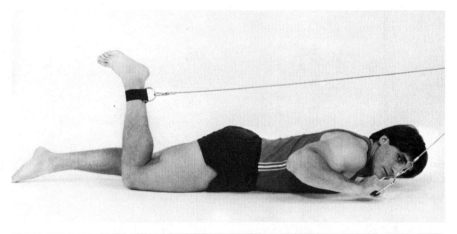

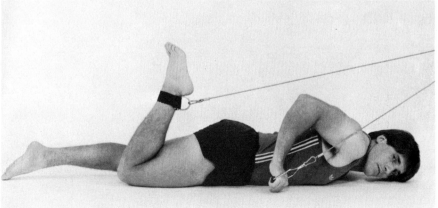

Hip Flexors

Attach the cable to the left leg, then lie flat on your stomach and face the pulley apparatus, holding the other end of the cable with the right hand.

Raise the left leg to a point of tightness.

Using the tightened hip muscles, attempt to drive the leg and knee back toward the floor, while slowly increasing the strength of the muscle contraction. The right hand holding the cable offers immovable resistance.

Hold for five seconds, exhale, and relax.

Raise the leg even higher to a new point of tightness, then repeat the exercise.

Do six repetitions, then switch to the other leg for six more.

Do not pull the leg higher with the pulley apparatus, but use the muscles in the leg and hips to raise the leg higher.

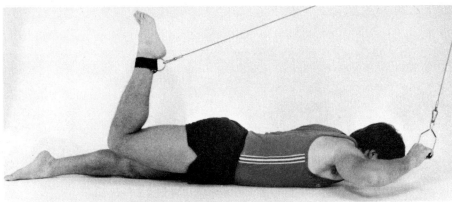

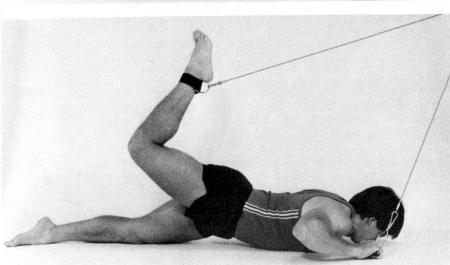

Groin

Attach one end of the cable apparatus to the left leg and hold the other end with the right hand. Spread the legs as far apart as possible to a point of tightness.

Using the groin muscles, try to pull the left knee back toward the right leg, while slowly increasing the strength of the muscle contraction. The pulley apparatus offers immovable resistance.

Hold for five seconds, exhale, and relax.

Open the left leg even farther to a new point of tightness, then repeat the exercise.

Do six repetitions, then switch to the other leg for six more.

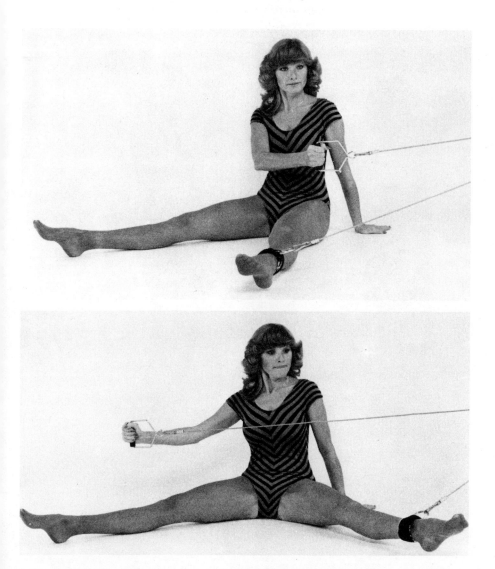

Shoulders

Attach the pulley close to the ground, then wrap the strap around the left wrist and raise the arm to a point of tightness, then bend the elbow to the back.

Hold the cable with the right hand at waist height.

Using the upper back (latissimus dorsi) muscles, attempt to pull the arm forward while slowly increasing the strength of the muscle contraction. The right hand on the cable offers immovable resistance.

Hold for five seconds, exhale, and relax.

Move the left arm farther to the rear to a new point of tightness, then repeat the exercise.

Do six repetitions, then switch to the other arm for six more.

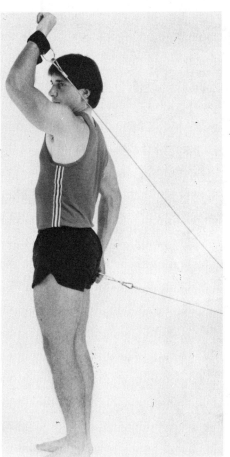 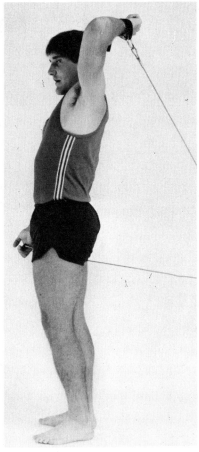

Attach the cable to the left wrist and hold the other end with the right hand, which is held high overhead. Move the left hand to a point of tightness at waist level.

Using the shoulder and chest muscles, attempt to pull the left arm back to the side of the left leg by slowly increasing the strength of the muscle contraction. The right hand on the other end of the cable apparatus offers immovable resistance.

Hold for five seconds, exhale, and relax.

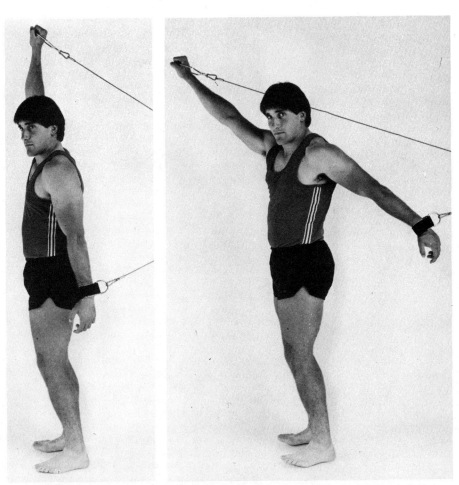

Move the left arm farther to the rear to a new point of tightness, then repeat the exercise.

Do six repetitions, then switch to the other arm for six more.

Attach the cable to the left wrist and hold the other end with the right hand. Stand with the back to the pulley apparatus and outstretch the arms to a point of tightness.

Move the left arm to the rear as much as possible at shoulder height.

Using the shoulder and chest muscles, attempt to swing the straight left arm back to the front while slowly increasing the strength of the muscle contractions. The right hand on the cable offers immovable resistance.

Hold for five seconds, exhale, and relax.

Move the left arm farther toward the rear to a new point of tightness, then repeat the exercise.

Do six repetitions, then switch to the other arm for six more.

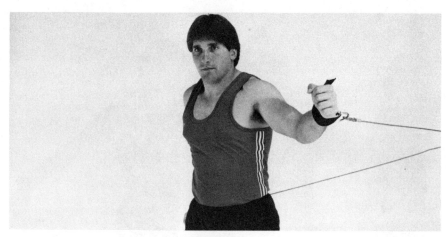

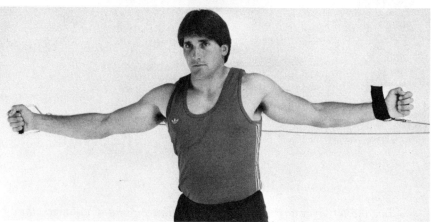

10

Relief for Chairbound Stiffness and Tension

We all get caught in positions of sitting or working where tensions gather and stiffness is a way of life.

The secretaries and office workers, long-distance travelers, assembly-line employees, students, housewives with a multitude of daily problems—name it and you can find people who get tense and sore.

Stretching isn't just for athletes. It applies to those in every walk of life. Included in this chapter are some suggested exercises for "chairbound" people who want to get rid of those tension headaches, sore backs, and stiff necks and shoulders.

These can be done every hour for a couple of minutes to relieve soreness and tension. Employers should encourage their employees to use them because they'll end up with healthier, happier workers.

Lower Back

Seated in a chair, pull both legs upward and attempt to touch your knees to your chest. Grasp your upper shins with both hands.

Pull your head toward your knees while also trying to squeeze your legs closer to your chest.

To increase the stretch, lean farther forward each time.

Pause after each repetition and exhale. Do six repetitions.

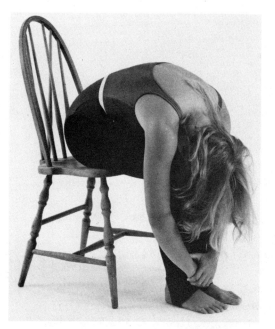
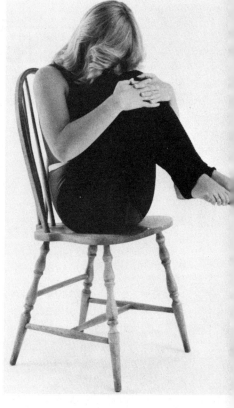

Seated in a chair, bend forward as far as possible so that your head touches your knees or reaches over them. Grasp your ankles with both hands and lower your head as far as possible.

To increase the stretch, gently pull yourself closer to the floor.

Pause after each repetition and exhale. Do six repetitions.

Seated upright in a chair, pull your right leg up to your chest and bend the knee as much as possible. Grasp the knee with both hands, then attempt to touch your chin to the knee, rolling your head forward.

To increase the stretch, bring the leg in closer to the chest.

Pause after each repetition and exhale. Do six repetitions, then switch to the other leg for six more.

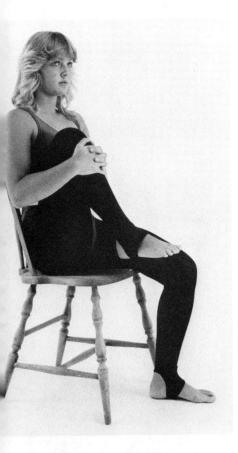

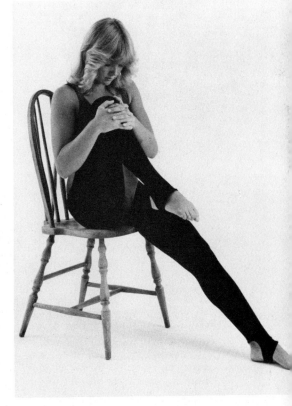

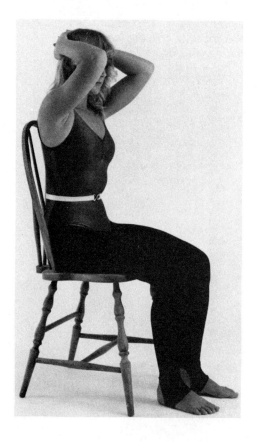

Shoulders

Sit upright in a chair and clasp your hands behind your head. Arch your back slightly, then pull your elbows backward like you are going to bring them together behind your head.

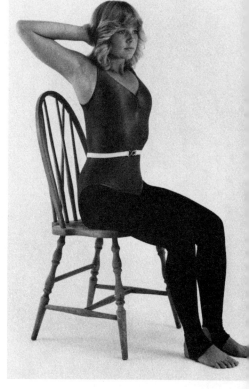

Pause after each repetition, exhale, relax the arms slightly, then stretch backward again. Do six repetitions.

This eases tension in the shoulders, opens the chest cavity for deeper breathing, and stretches the upper arm, back, and neck muscles.

This stretch will relieve tension in the neck and relax the shoulders.

Sitting upright, clasp your hands behind your head. Bend your head slightly forward, then try to touch your elbows to each other.

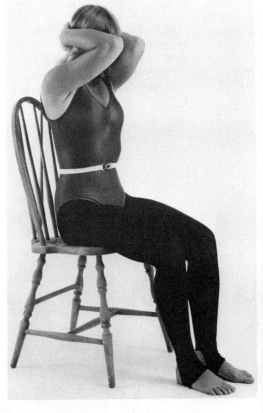

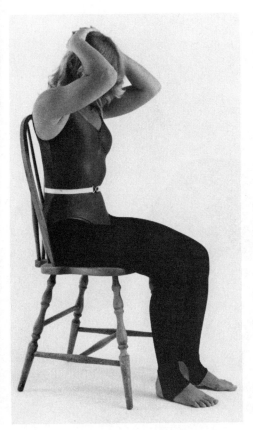

Pause and exhale. Sit back up and repeat the exercise, each time attempting to bring the elbows closer together. Do six repetitions.

Sides and Shoulders

Sit in a chair with good posture, then cross your right leg over your left. Reach around with your left hand and grasp the back of the chair. Put your right hand on the seat behind you as far to the left as possible.

Then turn as far as possible to the chair back.

To increase the stretch, reach farther behind the chair seat and turn farther.

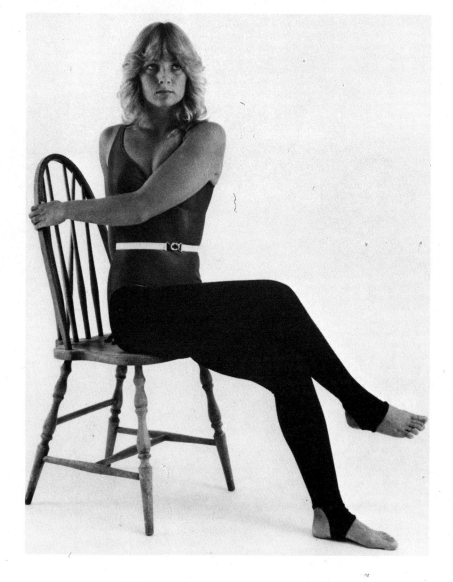

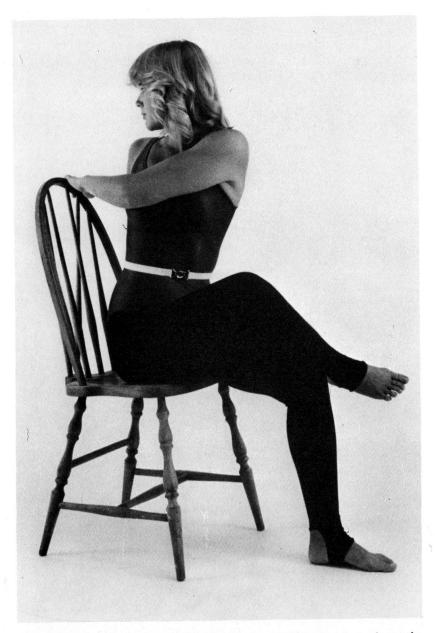

Pause each time and exhale. Do this six times, then reverse and turn the other way, crossing the left leg over the right and grasping the chair seat with the right hand, for six repetitions.

Shoulders

This exercise relieves tension in the upper back and shoulders.
Sit up straight in a chair and clasp your hands behind you. Then raise
your extended arms as high as possible.

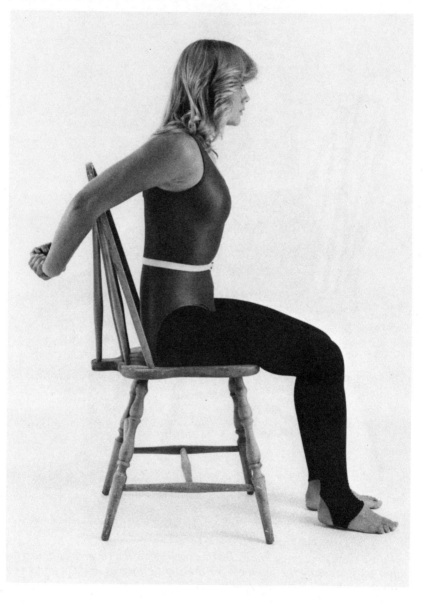

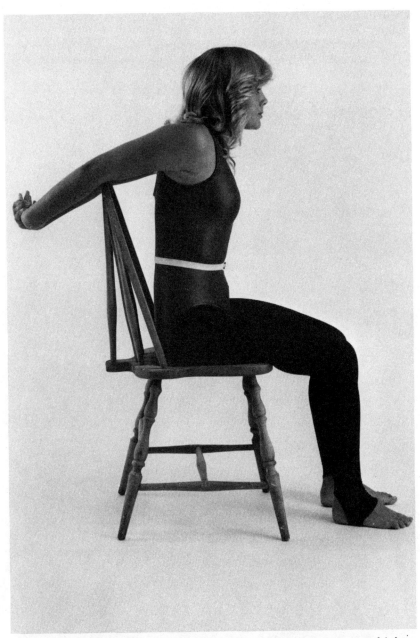

To increase the stretch, relax slightly, then raise your arms even higher. Pause after each repetition and exhale. Do six repetitions.

Sit as straight as possible in a chair and grasp the seat edges with your hands.

Holding on tightly, attempt to pull yourself into the seat with your fingers.

To increase the stretch, relax and then pull yourself even closer to the chair seat.

Pause after each repetition and exhale. Do this six times.

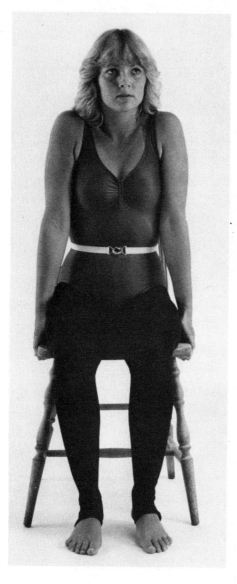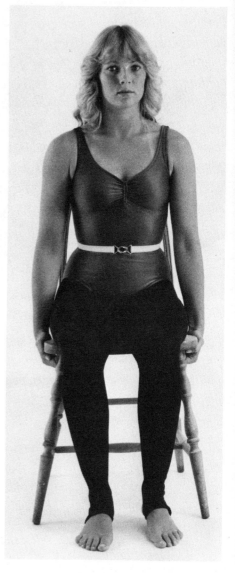

An easy way to release shoulder tension and open the chest for deeper breathing.

Sit up straight in a chair, then raise your hands as high as possible, lacing the fingers and turning the palms toward the ceiling.

To increase the stretch, try to reach a bit higher each time.

Pause after each repetition and exhale, relaxing. Do this six times.

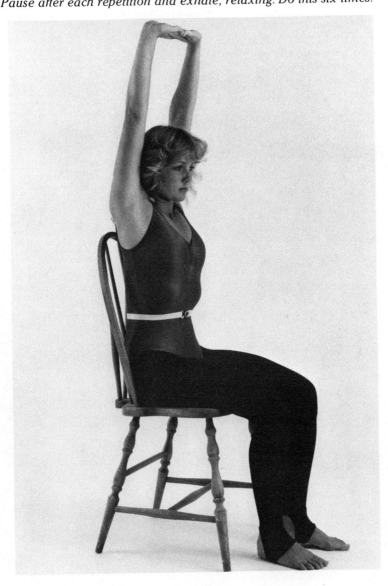

Neck

While sitting up straight, put your right hand behind your head and cup your chin in the left hand while your head is turned to the left to a point of tightness.

Using the neck muscles, push your chin toward the center, while slowly increasing the strength of the neck muscle contractions. Your hand will offer immovable resistance at the chin.

Hold for five seconds, exhale, and relax.

Turn your chin more toward your shoulder to a new point of tightness, then repeat the exercise.

Do six times, then switch hands, turn your head the other way, and repeat the sequence six times.

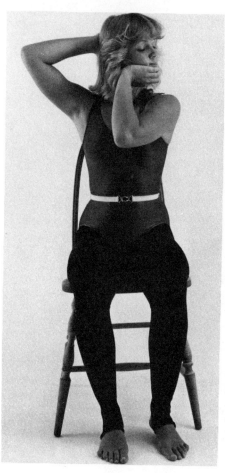 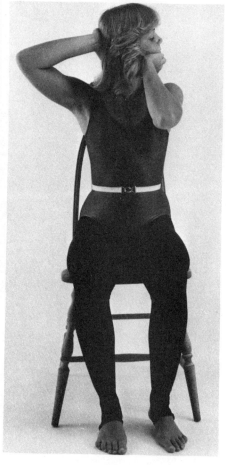

Shoulders and Back

Hold the chair seat with both hands and stretch out your feet as far as possible, holding your legs together and keeping the feet flat on the floor. In this arched position push your chest and abdomen upward and breathe very deeply.

To increase the stretch, arch upward more each time.

Pause after each repetition and exhale. Do six repetitions.

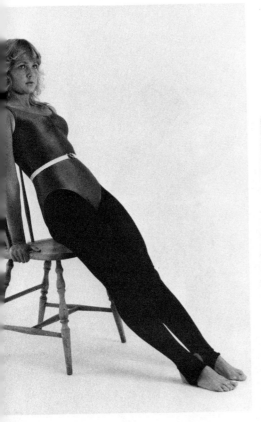
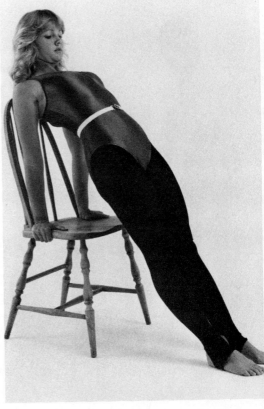

Shoulders

Sit in a chair and raise your arms behind you as far as possible. Have a partner lightly grasp your wrists.

Using the shoulder muscles, attempt to pull your arms forward, while slowly increasing the strength of the muscle contractions. Your partner's hands offer resistance to your wrists.

Hold for five seconds, exhale, and relax.

Move your arms farther to the rear, then repeat the exercise.

Do six repetitions.

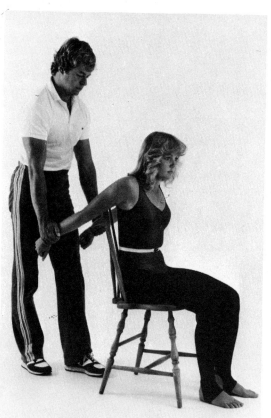
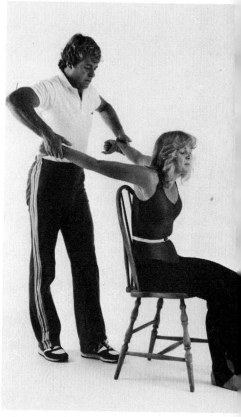

Raise your arms as high over your head as possible while sitting in your chair with good posture. Your partner should lightly grasp your wrists in his hands.

Tighten your shoulder muscles by reaching slightly behind you.

Slowly pull your arms forward while increasing the strength of the muscle contractions. Your partner's hands offer resistance.

Hold for five seconds, exhale, and relax.

Reach farther backward, then repeat the exercise.

Do six repetitions.

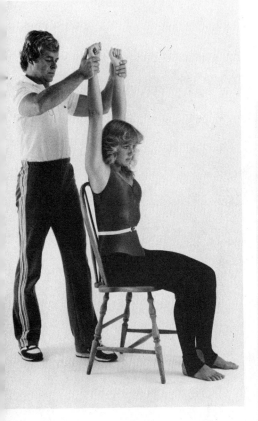
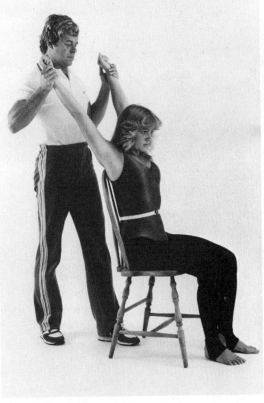

Shoulders

While sitting up straight, bend your arms and clasp your fingers behind your head, moving your arms to a point of tightness. Have your partner hold the inside of your elbows gently.

Pull your elbows forward as though you were going to touch them together in front of your face. Do this while slowly increasing the strength of the muscle contractions. Your partner's hands will offer immovable resistance.

Hold for five seconds, exhale, and relax.

Move your elbows farther backward to a new point of tightness, then repeat the exercise.

Do six repetitions.

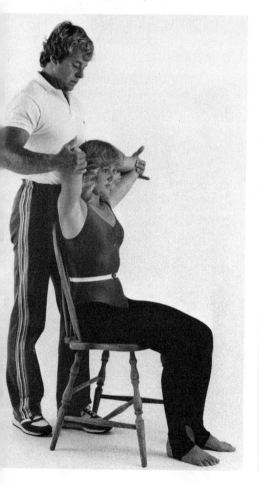
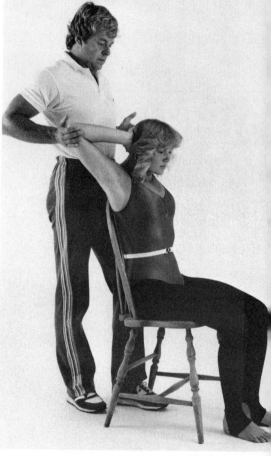

Neck

Sit upright and turn your head to the left to a point of tightness. Have a partner put one hand at the back of your head and cup your chin with the other hand.

Using the neck muscles, turn your head back toward your right while slowly increasing the strength of the neck muscle contractions. Your partner's hand on your chin will offer immovable resistance.

Hold for five seconds, exhale, and relax.

Turn your head farther to the left to a point of tightness, then repeat the exercise.

Do six times, then turn completely to the right and do six more times in the opposite direction.

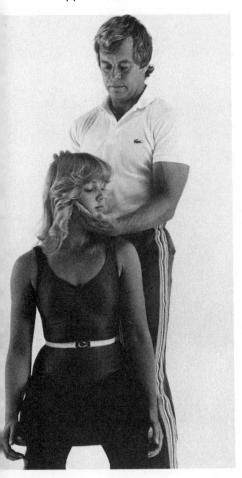
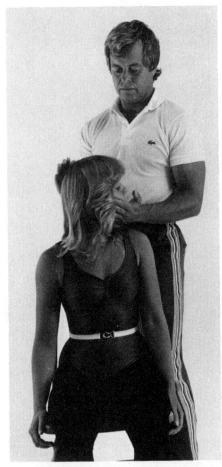

11

Racquet Sport Stretches

Weekend athletes are becoming more obsessed with racquet sports, such as racquetball, squash, and tennis, as recreational forms. These also lead to sore and torn muscles that hinder the participants for the next few days — injuries that can be avoided by a few minutes of simple stretching before engaging in the sports.

Racquet sports involve a lot of jumping, quick starts and stops, and arm swinging. Included here are some specific stretches that can be done at the court before beginning to hit warm-up shots.

Also look in the main part of the stretching portion of this book for ideas of other stretches that can be done if you can spend an extra few minutes before playing.

Stretch briefly after finishing to maintain some of the advantages you've gained from prestretching and playing.

Groin

Using the tennis racquet as a brace, stand up straight, spread your legs as far apart as possible, then turn to the right and reach out with the right foot pointed toward the tennis racquet.

The left foot stays pointed straight ahead and the heel is flat on the ground.

Lean your weight forward toward the racquet.

To increase the stretch, step even farther to the right and lean your weight farther forward.

Pause after each repetition and exhale. Do six repetitions, then switch and do six in the opposite direction.

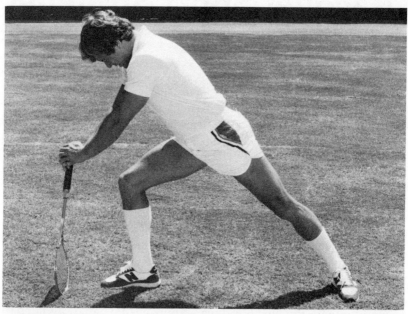

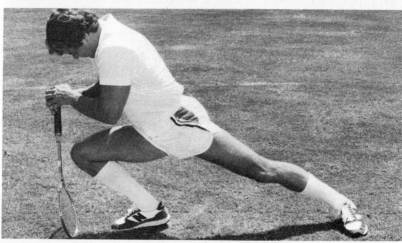

Lower Back

When lying down is inconvenient, try this stretch.

Stand up straight, then bend your right knee and move it as close as possible to your chest. Grasp the knee with both hands, then, pulling it tightly to the chest, attempt to touch it with your chin.

To increase the stretch, tighten the knee even more, get it closer to the chest, and bend your head farther forward.

Pause after each repetition and exhale. Do six repetitions, then switch and do six with the other leg.

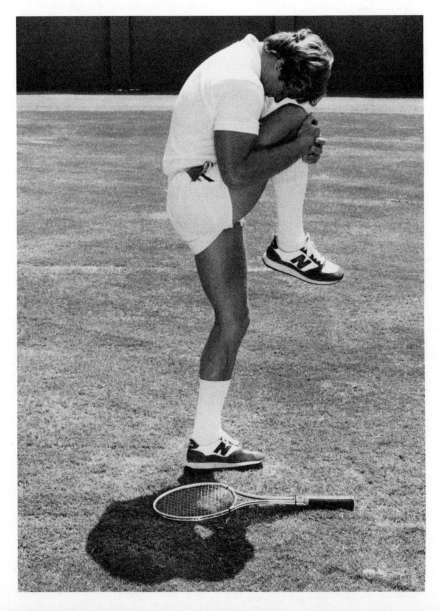

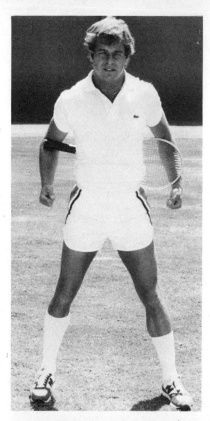

Sides and Shoulders

Hold the tennis racquet behind you with one arm looped over the handle and the other over the racquet's head. Turn as far to the right as possible, then reverse and turn slowly to the left. To increase the stretch, turn farther each time.

Pause in each repetition and exhale. Do six repetitions in each direction, pausing at each turn to get the full effect of the stretch.

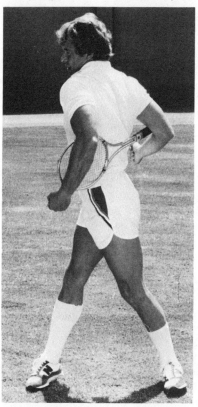

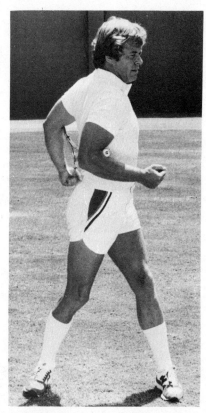

Shoulders

Hold the racquet as high overhead as possible, with both hands. Feet should be shoulder width apart. Then reach backward as far as possible with both hands.

To increase the stretch, reach farther backward each time.

Pause after each repetition and exhale. Do six repetitions.

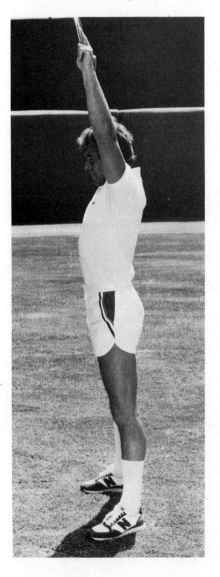
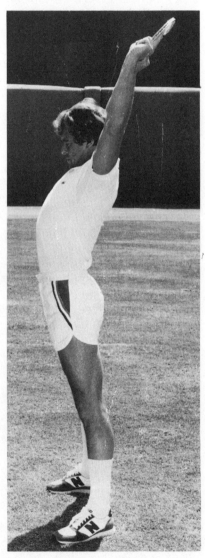

Shoulders and Lower Back

Stand with feet shoulder width apart and hold the racquet behind you with both hands at its ends. Keeping your arms extended, raise your hands as far as possible while standing up straight, then bend your upper body as if you are trying to reach the sky with your hands. To increase the stretch, reach higher and bend farther each time.

Pause after each repetition and exhale. Do six repetitions. Do not bounce your arms at the peak of this exercise.

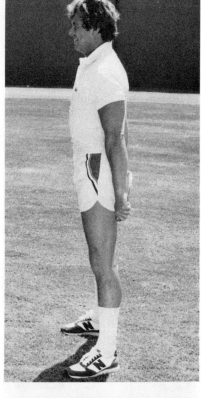

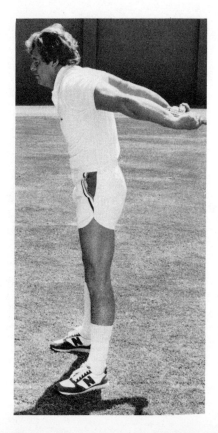

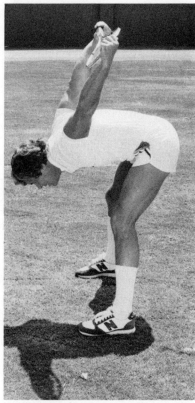

Shoulders and Sides

Hold the racquet behind you with it pointed, handle upward, at a 45 degree angle. Grasp the handle with the right hand and hold the head of the racquet with the left.

Pull the right hand backward with the left.

To increase the stretch, pull backward farther each time.

Hold at the peak for five seconds and breathe deeply. Exhale and relax. Do six repetitions, then reverse and hold the handle of the racquet with the left hand.

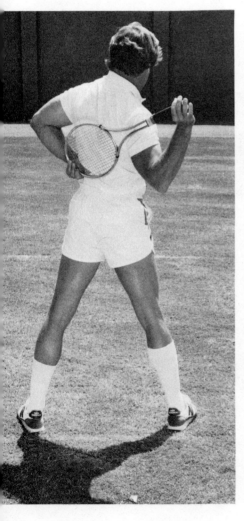
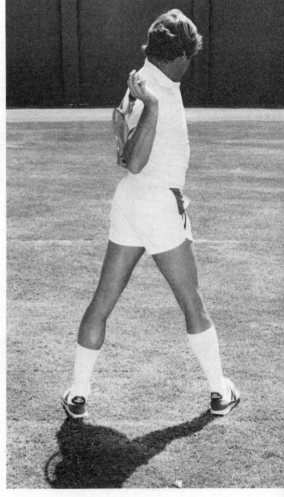

Triceps

Hold the racquet directly behind you with the handle pointing up, paralleling your spine. Grasp the handle with the right hand while holding the head of the racquet with the left.

Move the right arm backward to a point of tightness.

Using the upper back (latissimus dorsi) and tricep muscles, attempt to pull the racquet forward while your left hand offers resistance. Slowly increase the muscle contraction. This will cause the tricep muscle in the upper arm to stretch with some benefit to the shoulder and side.

Hold for five seconds, exhale, and relax.

Move the right arm backward to a new point of tightness, then repeat the exercise.

Do six repetitions, then reverse hand positions and do six more repetitions.

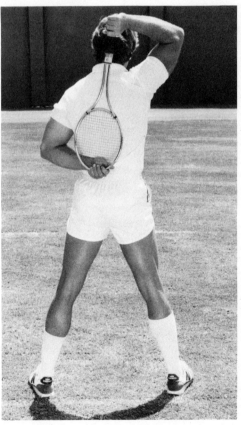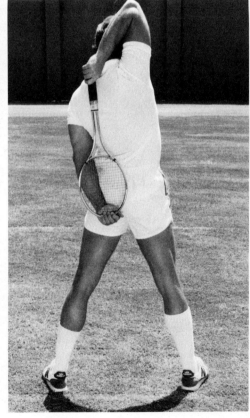

12

Golf, Baseball, Softball, and Hockey Stretches

Hitting a ball with a club or bat or a puck with a hockey stick involves more torso turning than most sports, so some exercises that can loosen up sides, shoulders, triceps muscles, and hip flexors have been included here for on-course or on-field warmups.

A lot of golfers and weekend softball players begin complaining about "bad backs." The stretches in this chapter may not save all the injuries, but they'll alleviate a lot of them.

They'll also make the swing flow a lot more easily because you'll be looser and more flexible. The shoulder turn in the golf swing will be enhanced, and the back should feel more comfortable.

After walking off the final green or swinging at the final pitch, take a couple of minutes to stretch again because potential soreness can be alleviated and flexibility gained from the poststretches.

Groin

Stand up straight and spread the legs as far apart as comfortable. Turn to the right and step forward as far as you can while keeping your left foot on the ground. Lean forward over the bent right knee as far as possible, always keeping the left foot flat.

To increase the stretch, lean farther forward each time.

Pause after each repetition and exhale. Do six repetitions, then switch and do six in the opposite direction.

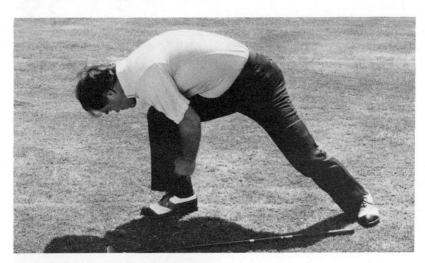

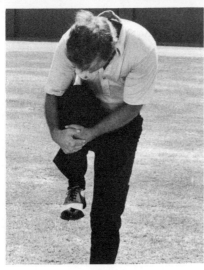

Lower Back

Stand up straight, then bend your right knee and move it as close as possible to your chest. Grasp the knee with both hands, then, pulling it tightly to the chest, attempt to touch it with your chin. To increase the stretch, bring your knee closer to the chest and bend your head farther forward.

Pause after each repetition and exhale. Do six repetitions, then switch and do six with the other leg.

Shoulders

Hold a golf club overhead as high as possible with both hands while your feet are spread at shoulder width. Then reach backward as far as possible.

To increase the stretch, reach farther backward each time.

Pause after each repetition and exhale. Do six times.

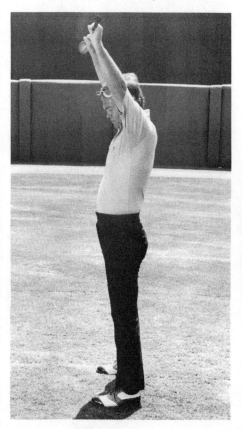
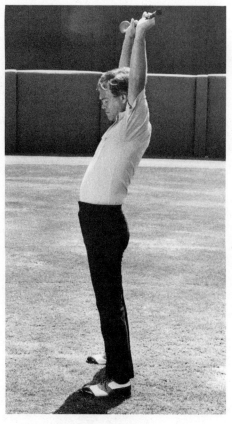

Shoulders and Lower Back

With feet spread at shoulder width, hold a golf club behind you with both hands gripping it near the ends. Keeping arms extended, raise them as high as possible while standing up straight.

Allow your upper body to bend forward at the waist as you reach as high as you can. To increase the stretch, reach higher each time.

Pause after each repetition and exhale. Do six repetitions. Do not bounce with your arms at the peak of this exercise.

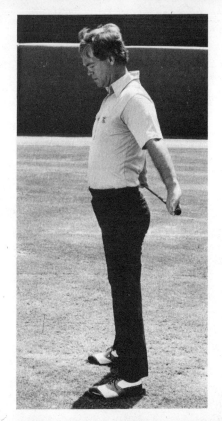

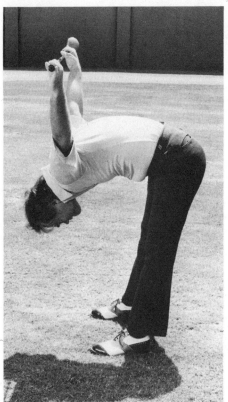

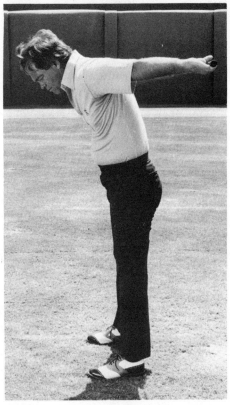

Triceps and Shoulders

Hold a golf club head in your left hand and grip the handle with your right hand over your head. Hold the club head forward with the left hand, which moves your right hand farther to the back.

To increase the stretch, progressively pull the club farther forward each time with the left hand.

Pause after each repetition and exhale. Do six times, then switch and hold the club head in the right hand and grasp the club grip with the left hand.

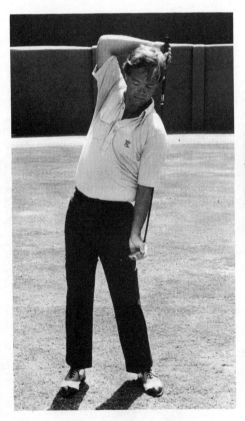
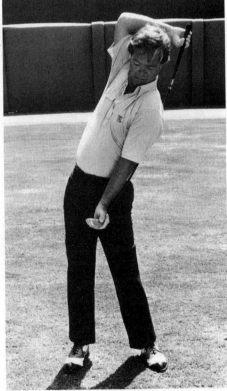

Sides

Hold a golf club across the back of your shoulders while standing up straight. Then use it as a lever to pull yourself as far as possible to the side. To increase the stretch, try to reach closer to the ground each time.

Pause after each repetition and exhale. Do six repetitions, alternating between touching to the left side and touching to the right.

It is important not to bend forward at the waist in this exercise to get the full effect.

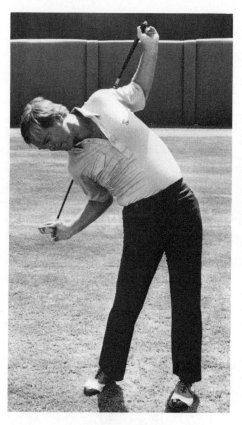

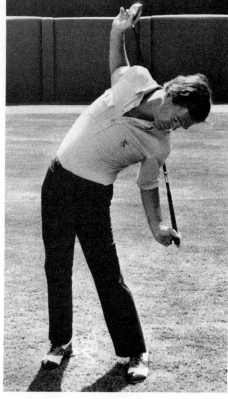

Lower Back and Sides

Hold a golf club across the broadest part of your back, bend forward at the waist, then pull the club head toward the ground as you twist your torso. To increase the stretch, twist farther each time.

Pause after each repetition and exhale. Do six repetitions, alternately turning to each side.

Do not bounce in this exercise.

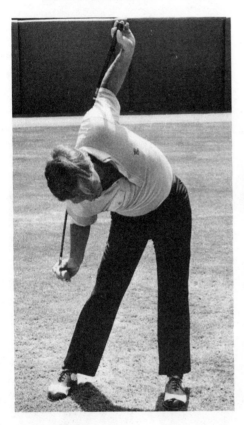
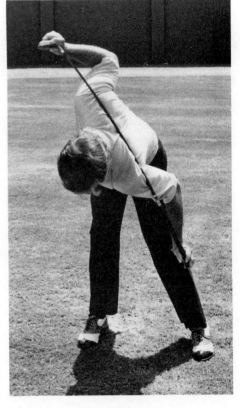

Side Twists

Hold a golf club across the broadest part of your shoulders and twist to the side. When you stop, use the hand on the golf club to pull yourself even farther.

To increase the stretch, pull yourself farther each time you twist.

Pause after each repetition and exhale. Do six repetitions, alternately turning to the left and to the right.

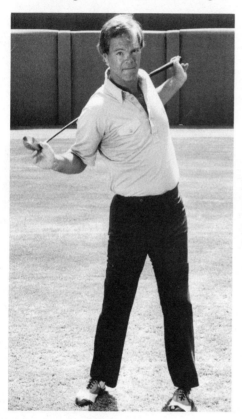

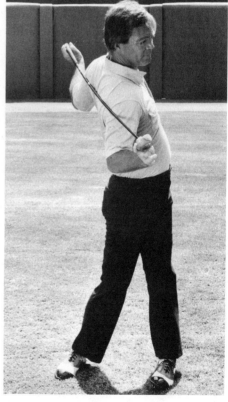

Hold a golf club across the middle of your back so that you can hook the handle end into one elbow. Hold the grip with your other hand, then turn as far as possible.

Use the hand on the grip to pull yourself into a new range of motion in the twist.

To increase the stretch, pull yourself farther into a turn each time.

Pause after each repetition and exhale. Do six times, then reverse the golf club and do six repetitions in the opposite direction.

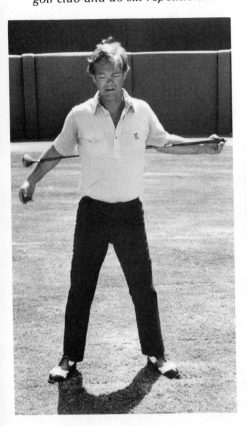

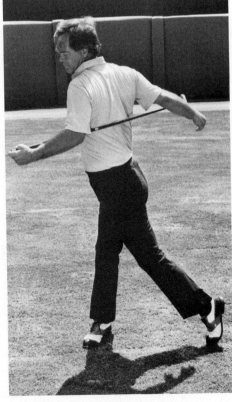

13

How the Pros Warm Up

Professional sports teams constantly are besieged with questions about stretching routines by coaches from colleges down to youth leagues.

The basic prepractice and pregame routine of the San Diego Chargers is included in this chapter. This stretching routine is applicable to all team-sports. Many players also will be stretched individually, especially those who do a lot of running, such as defensive backs, receivers, and running backs. Quarterbacks have their arms and shoulders worked on specifically.

Then all players meet on the field and go through the following exercises.

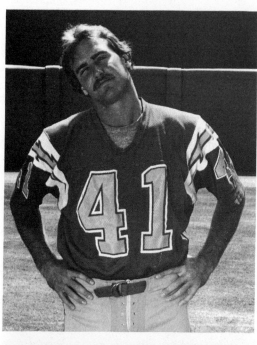

Neck

Slowly roll the head from side to side while standing up straight. Try to touch your chin to your chest on each rotation. At each shoulder, try progressively to touch your ear with the point of the shoulder.

Do not roll your head backward so that you are looking at the sky. This could cause some neck vertebrae problems.

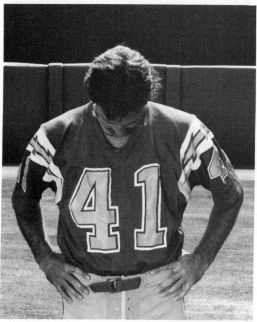

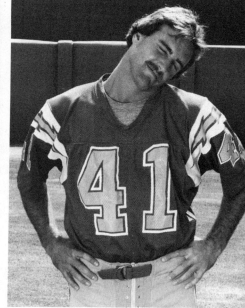

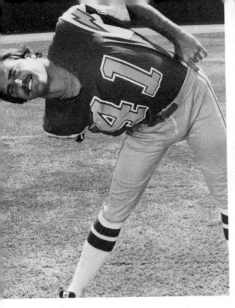
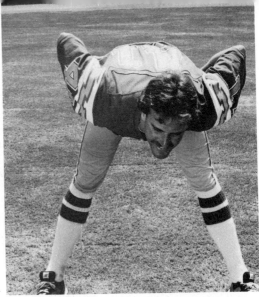

Trunk Twists

With legs slightly farther apart than shoulder width, put hands on waist, then stretch to one side. Move to a bent-forward position, reaching out as far as possible.

Stretch to the other side, bending at the side but not the waist. Then slowly roll to the back, reaching backward as far as is comfortable.

Do this six times, then reverse and do the twists in the opposite direction for another six repetitions.

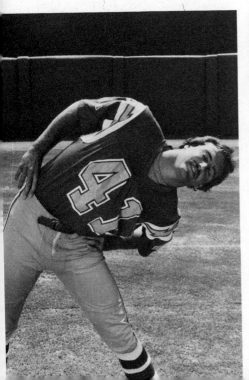
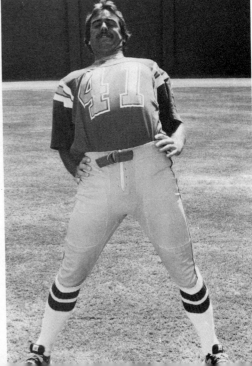

Torso Twists

With feet spread at shoulder width, turn to one side as far as possible. Then, using your hands and arms, reach as far behind you as possible. To increase the stretch, reach farther behind you each time.

Pause after each repetition and exhale. Do six times in each direction.

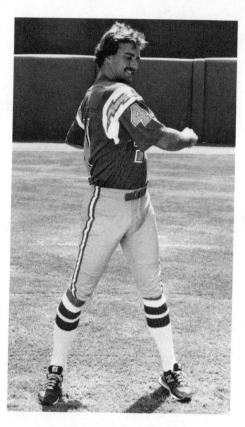

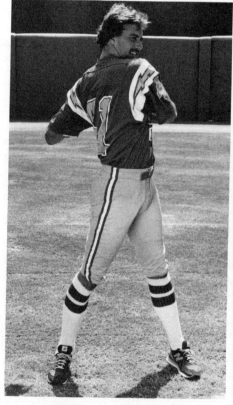

Groin and Hamstrings

Put your feet as far apart as possible. Slowly bend at the waist and reach for your right foot with both hands. Grasp your ankle, pause, then stand up straight again before reaching for the opposite leg.

To increase the stretch, reach farther down the leg each time.

Pause after each repetition and exhale. Do six repetitions in each direction.

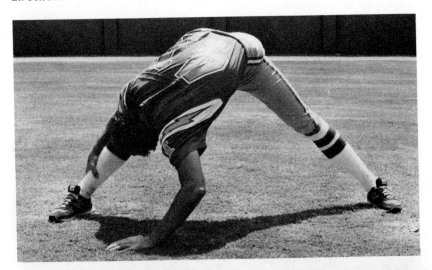

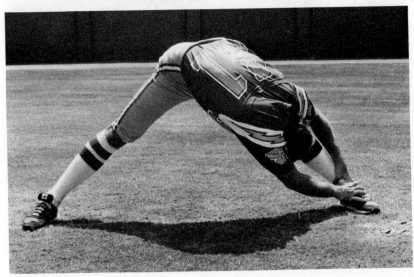

Groin

Stand up straight and spread feet as far apart as possible. Keeping your left foot pointed straight ahead, turn and stride to the right. Lean forward with your weight over your right knee. Keep your left foot flat on the ground.

To increase the stretch, lean farther forward and step farther to the right.

Pause after each repetition and exhale. Do six repetitions, then switch and do six in the opposite direction.

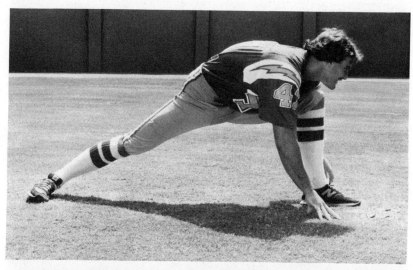

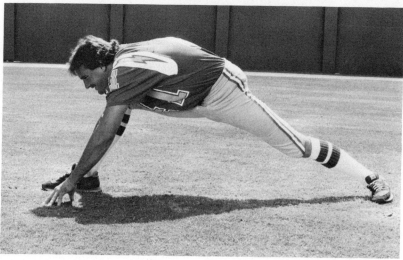

Thighs
(Quadriceps)

Lie on your stomach and bend your left leg backward to a point of tightness. Grasp the ankle with the left hand.

Using the tightened thigh muscle, try to force the foot back toward the ground while offering immovable resistance with your hand and slowly building muscle contraction.

Hold for five seconds, exhale, and relax.

Bend the leg farther to a new point of tightness, then repeat the exercise.

Do six repetitions, then switch to the right leg for six more.

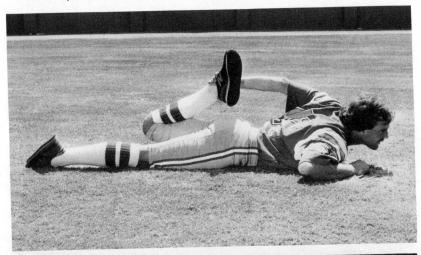

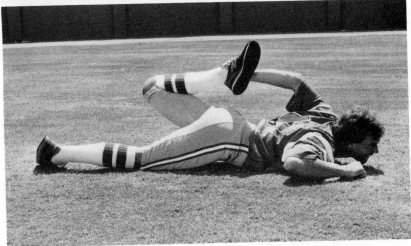

Groin and Hamstrings

Sit on the ground with legs outstretched and flat. Feet should be as far apart as possible. Reach for one foot, trying to grasp the ankle, and touch your forehead to your knee.

To increase the stretch, lean farther forward each time. You can also widen the area between your feet each time.

Pause after each repetition and exhale. Do six repetitions, then switch and do six with the other leg.

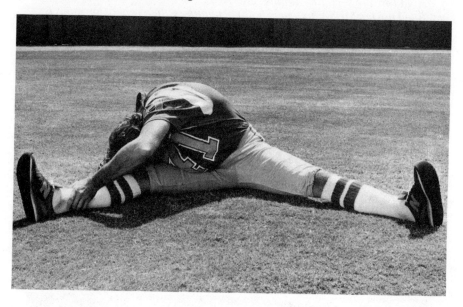

Hamstrings

Lie flat on your back on the ground and keep the left leg out straight at all times. Raise the right leg to a point of tightness, while keeping the knee straight. Grasp the right calf or ankle with both hands. Tighten the hamstring muscle.

Using the hamstring muscle, attempt to drive the heel back toward the ground while slowly increasing the strength of the muscle contraction. Your hands offer immovable resistance.

Hold for five seconds, exhale, and relax.

Move your leg farther back toward your head to a new point of tightness, then repeat the exercise.

Do six repetitions, then switch and do six with the other leg.

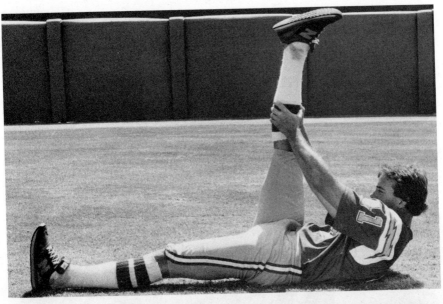

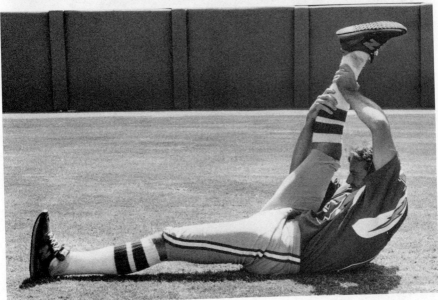

Lie flat on the ground, keeping the left leg stretched out straight. Raise the right knee to the chest and grasp the right leg across the hamstring with both arms.

Straighten the leg to a point of tightness.

Using the thigh muscles, attempt to straighten the leg even farther while slowly increasing the strength of the muscle contraction. Your hands offer immovable resistance.

Hold for five seconds, exhale, and relax.

Move your knee closer to your chest and attempt to straighten the leg out farther to a new point of tightness, as you repeat the exercise.

Do six repetitions, then switch to the other leg for six more.

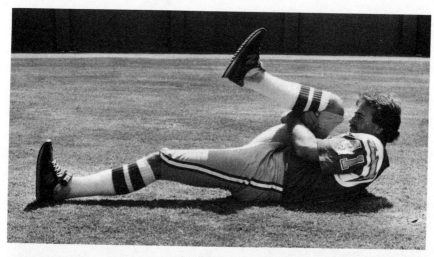

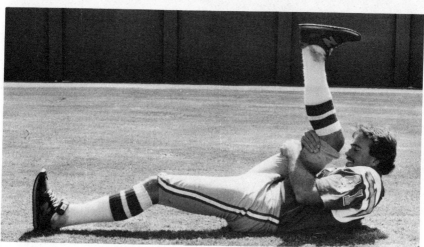

Lower Back

Pull both legs to the chest to a point of tightness while lying flat on the ground. Grasp the legs with both arms gripping around the hamstring muscles.

Using the lower back muscles, attempt to break the immovable grasp of the arms with your legs, while slowly increasing the strength of the muscle contraction. This will pull your head toward your knees and stretch the lower back.

Hold for five seconds, exhale, and relax.

Move your knees closer to your chest to a new point of tightness, then repeat the exercise.

Do six repetitions.

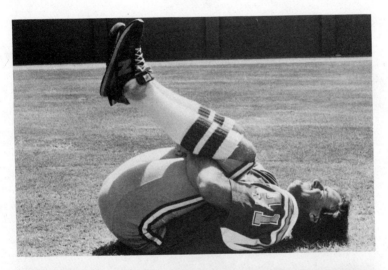

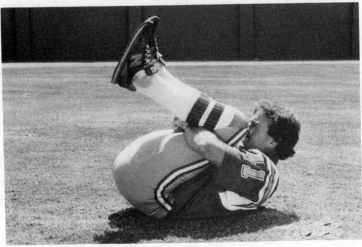

Groin

Sit with your legs as far apart as possible. Reach straight ahead to a point of tightness in the groin. Then lower your body toward the ground, trying to touch your elbows to the ground.

To increase the stretch, lean forward even more; also widen the area between your feet.

Pause after each repetition and exhale. Do six times.

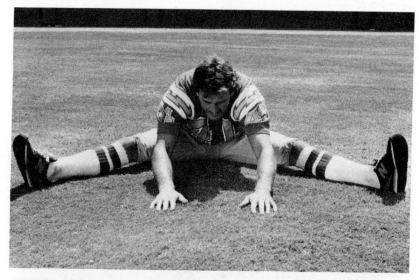

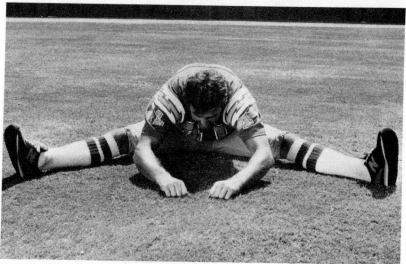

  Sit up straight and pull your feet together with your soles touching. When they are as close to your body as possible, lower your knees as close to the ground as is feasible.

  Rest your elbows along the inside of the lower legs.

  Using the groin muscles, attempt to push your knees together while slowly increasing the strength of the muscle contractions. Your elbows offer resistance.

  Hold for five seconds, exhale, and relax.

  Lower your knees closer to the ground and pull your feet closer to your body, then repeat the exercise. Do six repetitions.

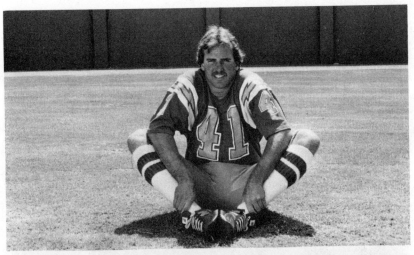

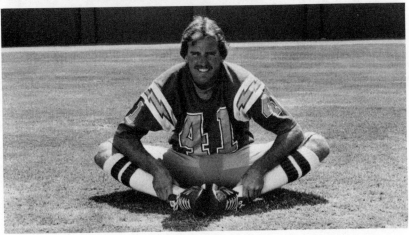

Hamstrings

Put your feet at shoulder width, then bend down so that your hands are six inches from the feet with the knees touching your chest. Slowly straighten up fully, feeling the stretch in the hamstring area.

To increase the stretch, move your hands closer to your feet.

Pause after each repetition and exhale. Do six repetitions.

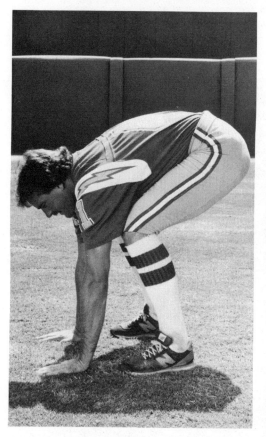

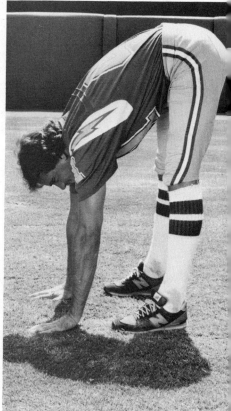

Hamstrings and Hip Flexors

Stretch out fully on the ground on your back, then move the left leg across the right so that the right hand can grasp the left ankle. Keep both shoulders flat on the ground.

To increase the stretch, move the leg up farther toward the left shoulder.

Pause after each repetition and exhale. Do six repetitions, then switch to the other leg for six more.

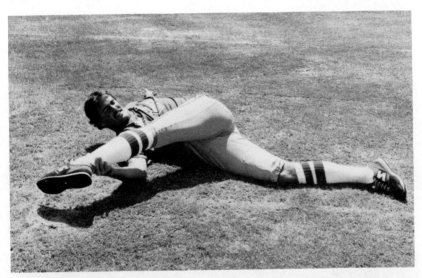

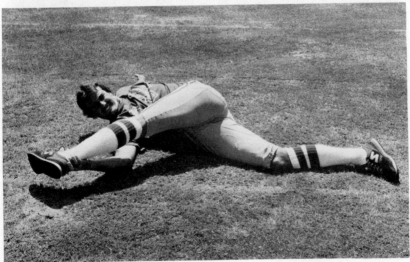

Hip Flexors

Lie on your side, lift the top leg, and bend the knee as far as it will go. Grasp the ankle with your hand and move it backward to a point of tightness.

Using the hip muscles, attempt to pull the leg out of your grasp while slowly increasing the strength of the muscle contraction. Your hand offers immovable resistance.

Hold for five seconds, exhale, and relax.

Raise the leg farther to a new point of tightness, then repeat the exercise.

Do six repetitions, then switch to the other leg for six more.

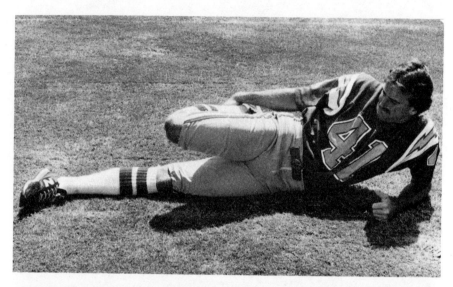

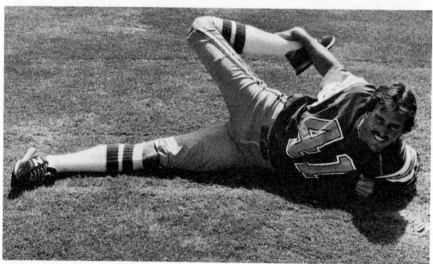

Appendix
Stretches by Body Part

STRETCHES FOR THE SHOULDERS:
pages 21-22, 57-58, 76, 94, 96-97, 105, 120-22, 126-33, 135-38, 144-47, 151-53

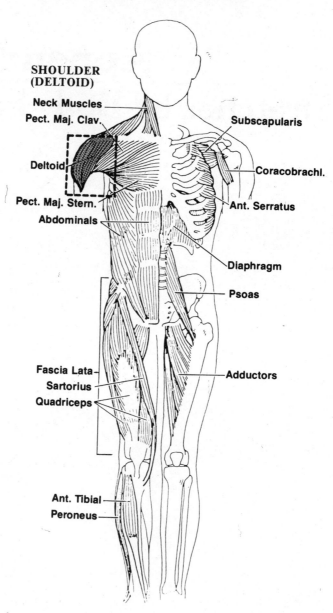

STRETCHES FOR THE CHEST:
page 95

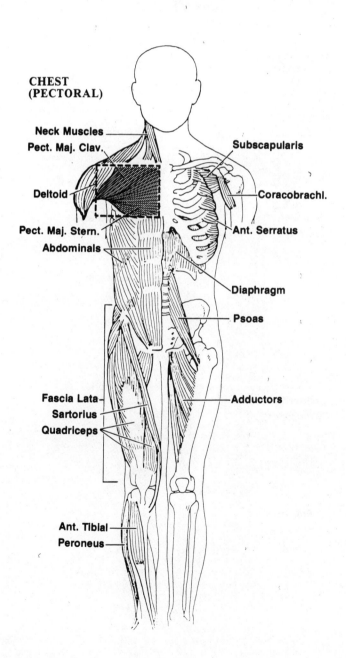

CHEST
(PECTORAL)

Neck Muscles
Pect. Maj. Clav.
Deltoid
Pect. Maj. Stern.
Abdominals
Fascia Lata
Sartorius
Quadriceps
Ant. Tibial
Peroneus

Subscapularis
Coracobrachi.
Ant. Serratus
Diaphragm
Psoas
Adductors

STRETCHES FOR THE SHOULDERS AND CHEST:
page 21

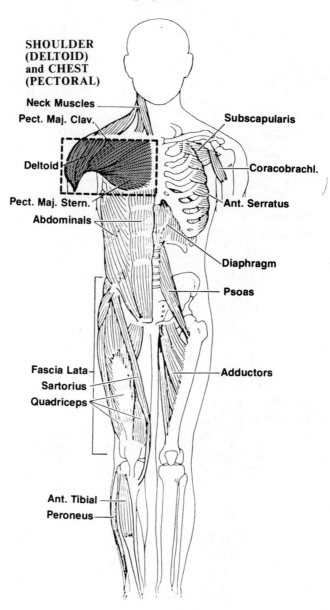

SHOULDER
(DELTOID)
and CHEST
(PECTORAL)

Neck Muscles

Pect. Maj. Clav.

Subscapularis

Deltoid

Coracobrachl.

Pect. Maj. Stern.

Ant. Serratus

Abdominals

Diaphragm

Psoas

Fascia Lata

Sartorius

Quadriceps

Adductors

Ant. Tibial

Peroneus

STRETCHES FOR THE TRUNK:
pages 32, 161

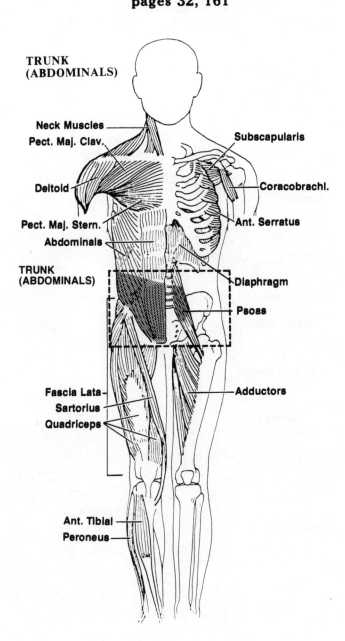

TRUNK
(ABDOMINALS)

Neck Muscles
Pect. Maj. Clav.

Subscapularis

Deltoid

Coracobrachi.

Pect. Maj. Stern.

Ant. Serratus

Abdominals

TRUNK
(ABDOMINALS)

Diaphragm

Psoas

Fascia Lata
Sartorius
Quadriceps

Adductors

Ant. Tibial
Peroneus

STRETCHES FOR THE UPPER BACK:
pages 52, 73, 99-100, 113, 130-31, 135

**UPPER BACK
(POSTERIOR
DELTOIDS,
TRAPEZIUS,
LATISSIMUS
DORSI)**

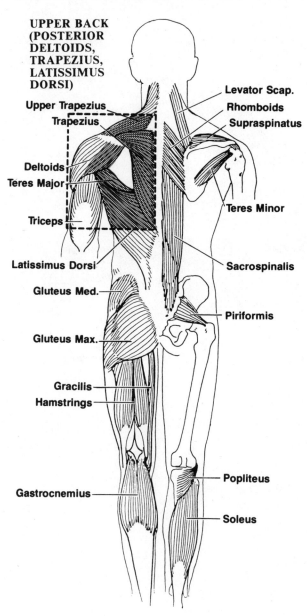

Upper Trapezius
Trapezius

Deltoids
Teres Major

Triceps

Latissimus Dorsi

Gluteus Med.

Gluteus Max.

Gracilis
Hamstrings

Gastrocnemius

Levator Scap.
Rhomboids
Supraspinatus

Teres Minor

Sacrospinalis

Piriformis

Popliteus

Soleus

STRETCHES FOR THE
LOWER BACK:

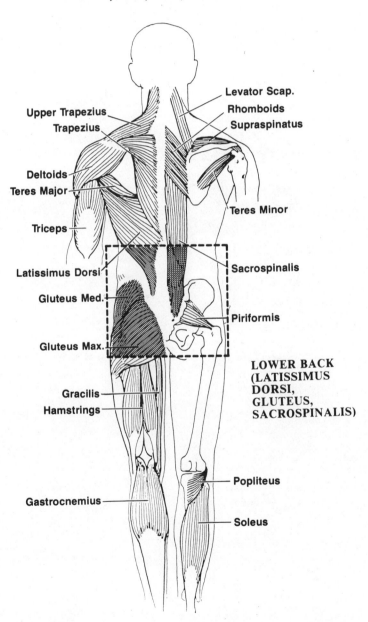

Levator Scap.
Rhomboids
Supraspinatus

Upper Trapezius
Trapezius

Deltoids
Teres Major

Teres Minor

Triceps

Latissimus Dorsi

Sacrospinalis

Gluteus Med.

Piriformis

Gluteus Max.

**LOWER BACK
(LATISSIMUS
DORSI,
GLUTEUS,
SACROSPINALIS)**

Gracilis
Hamstrings

Popliteus

Gastrocnemius

Soleus

STRETCHES FOR THE SIDES:
pages 49-51, 71, 92-93, 112, 128-29, 144, 147, 154-55, 156-57

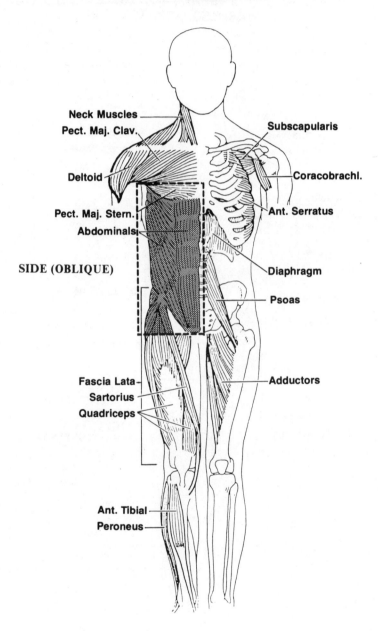

Neck Muscles
Pect. Maj. Clav.
Subscapularis
Deltoid
Coracobrachl.
Pect. Maj. Stern.
Ant. Serratus
Abdominals
SIDE (OBLIQUE)
Diaphragm
Psoas
Fascia Lata
Sartorius
Quadriceps
Adductors
Ant. Tibial
Peroneus

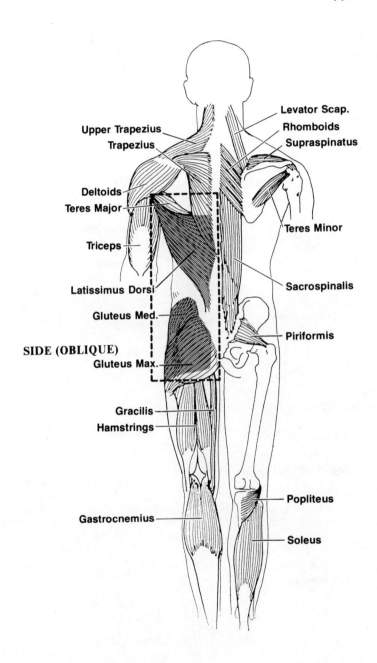

Levator Scap.
Rhomboids
Supraspinatus
Upper Trapezius
Trapezius
Deltoids
Teres Major
Teres Minor
Triceps
Latissimus Dorsi
Sacrospinalis
Gluteus Med.
Piriformis
SIDE (OBLIQUE)
Gluteus Max.
Gracilis
Hamstrings
Popliteus
Gastrocnemius
Soleus

STRETCHES FOR THE THIGHS:
pages 45-47, 66-67, 83, 88-89, 110, 117, 165

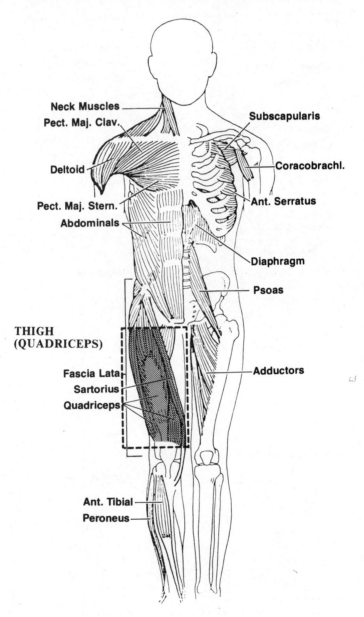

Neck Muscles

Pect. Maj. Clav.

Subscapularis

Deltoid

Coracobrachl.

Pect. Maj. Stern.

Ant. Serratus

Abdominals

Diaphragm

Psoas

THIGH
(QUADRICEPS)

Fascia Lata

Sartorius

Quadriceps

Adductors

Ant. Tibial

Peroneus

STRETCHES FOR THE HAMSTRINGS:
pages 4-5, 14, 18, 41-44, 64-65, 81-82, 91, 109, 115-16, 163, 166-68, 172-73

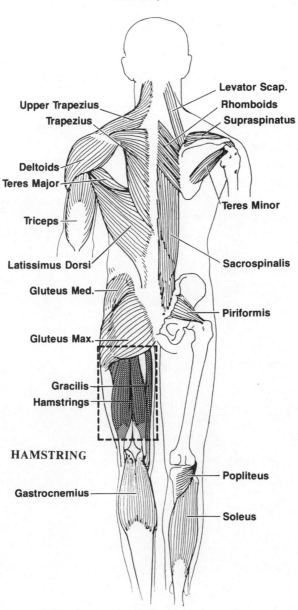

Upper Trapezius

Trapezius

Deltoids

Teres Major

Triceps

Latissimus Dorsi

Gluteus Med.

Gluteus Max.

Gracilis

Hamstrings

HAMSTRING

Gastrocnemius

Levator Scap.

Rhomboids

Supraspinatus

Teres Minor

Sacrospinalis

Piriformis

Popliteus

Soleus

STRETCHES FOR THE SHINS:
pages 39-40, 64, 80

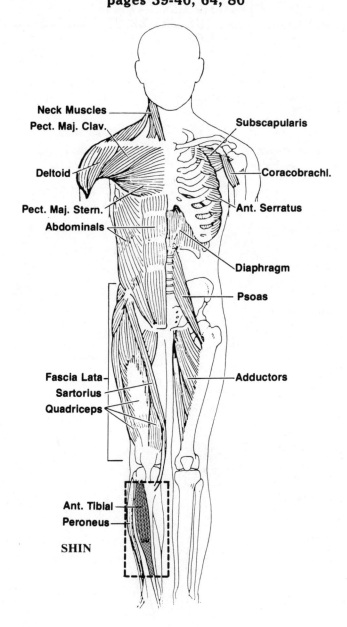

Neck Muscles

Pect. Maj. Clav.

Subscapularis

Deltoid

Coracobrachi.

Pect. Maj. Stern.

Ant. Serratus

Abdominals

Diaphragm

Psoas

Fascia Lata

Adductors

Sartorius

Quadriceps

Ant. Tibial

Peroneus

SHIN

STRETCHES FOR THE CALVES AND ACHILLES TENDONS:
pages 38-39, 62-63, 80, 108-9

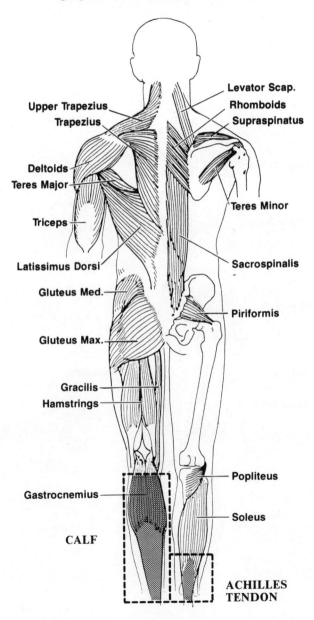

Levator Scap.
Rhomboids
Supraspinatus
Upper Trapezius
Trapezius
Deltoids
Teres Major
Teres Minor
Triceps
Latissimus Dorsi
Sacrospinalis
Gluteus Med.
Piriformis
Gluteus Max.
Gracilis
Hamstrings
Popliteus
Gastrocnemius
Soleus
CALF
ACHILLES TENDON

STRETCHES FOR THE HIP FLEXORS:
pages 21, 68-70, 84, 88-89, 111, 118, 173-74

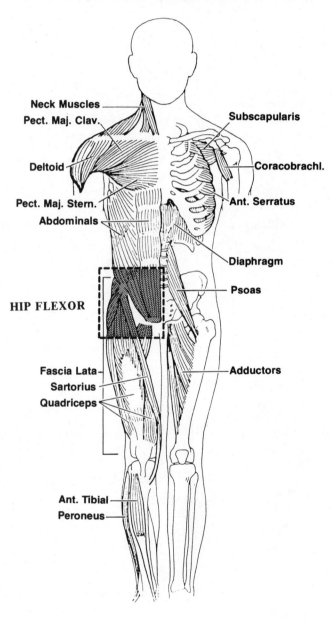

Neck Muscles
Pect. Maj. Clav.
Deltoid
Pect. Maj. Stern.
Abdominals

Subscapularis
Coracobrachl.
Ant. Serratus
Diaphragm
Psoas

HIP FLEXOR

Fascia Lata
Sartorius
Quadriceps

Adductors

Ant. Tibial
Peroneus

STRETCHES FOR THE GROIN:
pages 22, 47-49, 74-75, 85, 91, 119, 142, 150, 163-64, 166, 170-71

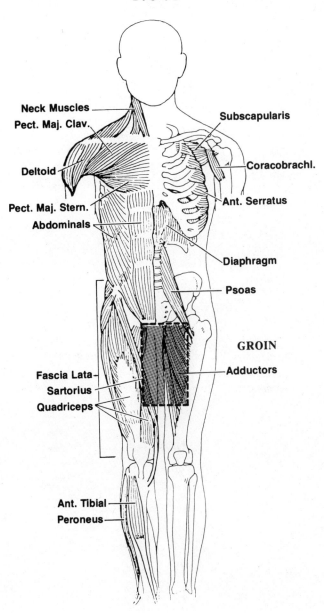

Neck Muscles

Pect. Maj. Clav.

Subscapularis

Deltoid

Coracobrachl.

Pect. Maj. Stern.

Ant. Serratus

Abdominals

Diaphragm

Psoas

GROIN

Fascia Lata

Adductors

Sartorius

Quadriceps

Ant. Tibial

Peroneus

STRETCHES FOR THE NECK:
pages 26, 59-60, 77-78, 103-4, 134, 139, 160

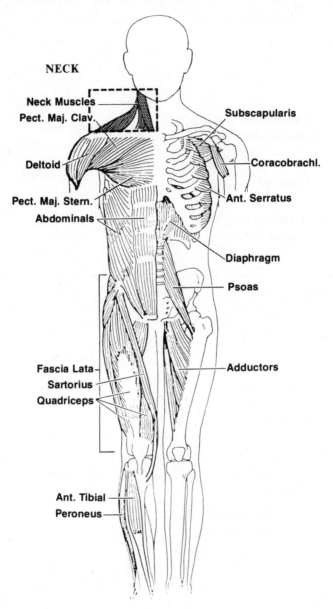

NECK

Neck Muscles
Pect. Maj. Clav.

Deltoid

Pect. Maj. Stern.

Abdominals

Fascia Lata
Sartorius
Quadriceps

Ant. Tibial
Peroneus

Subscapularis

Coracobrachl.

Ant. Serratus

Diaphragm

Psoas

Adductors

STRETCHES FOR THE TRICEPS:
pages 98, 148, 153

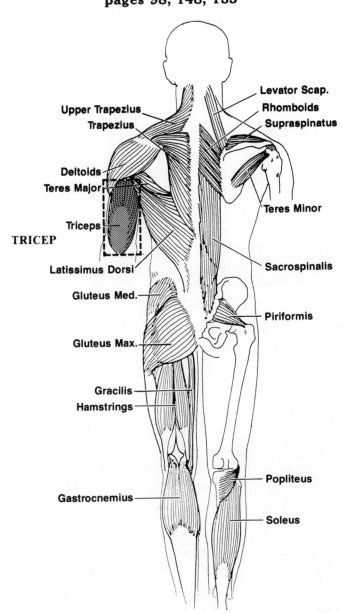

Upper Trapezius

Trapezius

Deltoids

Teres Major

Triceps

TRICEP

Latissimus Dorsi

Gluteus Med.

Gluteus Max.

Gracilis

Hamstrings

Gastrocnemius

Levator Scap.

Rhomboids

Supraspinatus

Teres Minor

Sacrospinalis

Piriformis

Popliteus

Soleus

Bibliography

Asmussen, E., and Boje, O. "Body Temperature and Capacity for Work," *Acta Physiologic Scandanavia.* 10:1-22, 1945.

Astrand, Per Olof, *Work Physiology.* New York: McGraw-Hill, 1970.

Crutchfield, Carolyn A., Barnes, Marylou R., *The Neurophysiological Basis of Patient Treatment.* 1973.

DeVries, Herbert A., *Physiology of Exercises,* Dubuque, IA: William C. Brown Co., 1977.

Index

195